Research-focused Careers for Paramedics

Research-focused Careers for Paramedics

Edited by

Gregory A. Whitley

School of Health and Care Sciences
University of Lincoln
Lincoln, United Kingdom

Clinical Audit and Research Unit
East Midlands Ambulance
Service NHS Trust
Lincoln, United Kingdom

Scott Munro

School of Health Sciences
University of Surrey
Guildford, United Kingdom

Nexus House
South East Coast Ambulance
Service NHS Trust
Crawley, United Kingdom

WILEY

This edition first published 2025
© 2025 John Wiley & Sons Ltd

Registered Offices
John Wiley & Sons, Inc., 111 River Street, Hoboken, NJ 07030, USA
John Wiley & Sons Ltd, New Era House, 8 Oldlands Way, Bognor Regis, West Sussex, PO22 9NQ, UK

For details of our global editorial offices, customer services, and more information about Wiley products visit us at www.wiley.com.

The manufacturer's authorized representative according to the EU General Product Safety Regulation is Wiley-VCH GmbH, Boschstr. 12, 69469 Weinheim, Germany, e-mail: Product_Safety@wiley.com.

Wiley also publishes its books in a variety of electronic formats and by print-on-demand. Some content that appears in standard print versions of this book may not be available in other formats.

Library of Congress Cataloging-in-Publication Data Applied for
Paperback ISBN: 9781394241248

Cover Design: Wiley
Cover Images: © The img/Shutterstock, © Yellow_man/Shutterstock

Set in 11.5/14pt STIX Two Text by Straive, Pondicherry, India

Contents

About the Contributors

Alan Michael Batt, PhD
Alan is an Associate Professor (adjunct) at Monash University, the Paramedicine Programme Lead and an Assistant Professor (adjunct) at Queen's University, and an Assistant Professor (status) at the University of Toronto. He originally qualified as a paramedic in Ireland and has since gained experience in nine countries across four continents. He is a Co-Chair of the McNally Project for Paramedicine Research in Canada, a Fellow of the Higher Education Academy (United Kingdom), and a Member of the Academy of Medical Educators (United Kingdom). Alan's programme of research uses mixed methods approaches to explore health professions education, with a focus on professional competencies, the evolving role of paramedicine, care of

marginalised populations, and social and structural determinants of health. He is a Deputy Editor of *Paramedicine* and serves as a Senior Appraiser with the Prehospital Evidence-Based Practice Project at Dalhousie University. He has published over 190 articles, reports, and chapters and has presented at international and national conferences on more than 200 occasions. His research has attracted over $3.7m CAD in research funding, and he has received multiple awards for his scholarly and professional contributions to paramedicine.

Malcolm Boyle, PhD

Malcolm is an Associate Professor and an Academic Lead in Paramedic Education and a Programme Director for Paramedicine Programmes at Griffith University. He was a paramedic for over 35 years, with the last 28 years as a Mobile Intensive Care Ambulance (MICA) Paramedic in Victoria, primarily working in rural areas. He has been working in academia since 1999 and moved to Griffith University in July 2016, prior to that he was at Monash University in Melbourne, Australia. Malcolm's PhD research focused on triage and error detection in pre-hospital trauma management. Malcolm is a Fellow of the Australasian College of Paramedicine, and he has published over 200 academic outputs and secured over $2.5m AUD in research funding as a chief investigator or co-applicant.

Georgette Eaton, DPhil (Oxon)

Georgette is the Consultant Paramedic in Urgent Care at London Ambulance Service NHS Trust and an Honorary Researcher at the Nuffield Department of Primary Care Health Sciences at the University of Oxford. Georgette completed her DPhil (PhD) in Evidence-Based Health Care at the University of Oxford in 2024, where her research —funded by a Doctoral Research Fellowship from the National Institute for Health and Care Research—explored the impact of paramedics in NHS primary care, using realist approaches to improve understanding, support intelligent policy, and make recommendations for future workforce planning. Georgette is a facilitator and co-chair within the Oxfordshire Community for Allied Health Professions Research, as well as a Scientist International Collaborator in the McNally Project and a Deputy Editor for *Paramedicine*.

Ben Meadley, PhD
Ben Meadley is an Intensive Care Paramedic and the Director of Paramedicine at Ambulance Victoria. He is a registered paramedic who commenced his career with Ambulance Victoria in 1998, followed by a period with New South Wales Ambulance from 1999 to 2003. Returning to Ambulance Victoria, Ben trained as an intensive care (MICA) paramedic in 2004 and an intensive care (MICA) flight paramedic in 2009. He joined the staff of Monash University in 2003, and he has held the positions of Teaching Associate, Lecturer, and Unit Coordinator in the undergraduate and postgraduate programmes. Ben completed his PhD at Monash Paramedicine, investigating the physiological and metabolic health of paramedics, as well as human performance in specialist teams. Ben has developed expertise in pre-hospital critical care, paramedic education, human performance, and paramedic health and well-being. His research interests include respiratory and cardiovascular physiology, point-of-care ultrasound, human performance optimisation, and selection to specialist paramedicine teams. Ben divides his time

between clinical, teaching, and research roles. He is also a Fellow of the Australasian College of Paramedicine and was awarded the Ambulance Service Medal in 2023.

Elisha Miller, MSc

Elisha's career in the ambulance service began as an urgent call taker in the Yorkshire Ambulance Service NHS Trust (YAS) control room. With a desire to advance clinically, she applied for the paramedic science programme at Coventry University, graduating as a paramedic in 2013. She then served as an operational paramedic for West Midlands Ambulance Service University NHS Foundation Trust until March 2016, when she relocated back to Yorkshire to work as a frontline paramedic. In October 2019, she joined the YAS Research and Development team as a Research Paramedic, where she assisted in leading the delivery of the YAS research portfolio, including successfully applying for College of Paramedics small grants to fund her own research study.

In 2020, Elisha presented the findings from her Advanced Clinical Practice MSc dissertation at the College of Paramedics' Fourth Annual National Research Conference, where her abstract was published in the *British Paramedic Journal*, and her full paper is currently awaiting publication. In December 2023, she obtained an 18-month secondment to the National Institute for Health and Care Research Academy as a Senior Programme Manager, overseeing funding programmes that support health and social care professionals in their clinical and academic careers. Alongside this role, she is due to complete her MSc in Clinical Research Delivery at the University of Sheffield in 2025 and serves as a reviewer for the *British Paramedic Journal*.

Brendan Shannon, PhD

Brendan is an Associate Professor and the Deputy Head of the Department of Paramedicine at Monash University and a member of the Australasian College of Paramedicine Community Paramedicine working group. A registered paramedic with more than a decade of clinical experience, Brendan is passionate about refining healthcare models to ensure underserved communities receive the requisite care and support. He is known for innovating new education programmes and paramedicine models of care and career pathways that facilitate this, including as the Education Lead for the Victorian Paramedic Practitioner programme. Brendan's doctoral research focused on the impact of health services implementing alternative care pathways in community settings. As a health services researcher, he has published extensively, demonstrating his commitment to translating complex data into actionable insights to enhance healthcare delivery and patient outcomes. Brendan's collaborative, data-driven approach has earned him domestic and international recognition, which he applies to his own research and teaching, as well as the research he supervises.

Peter O'Meara, PhD

Peter is an internationally recognised expert on paramedicine models of care and education. He is an Adjunct Professor of Paramedicine at Monash and Charles Sturt Universities in Australia, a Board Member of the Paramedic Network and the American Paramedic Association in the United States, a Fellow of the Australasian College of Paramedicine, and a member of several national and international advisory committees. His academic studies have been diverse and encompass health administration, public policy, and agricultural health and medicine.

Peter is a well-published and cited paramedic author of more than 100 peer-reviewed papers as well as several book chapters, and innumerable commentaries and editorials. He has examined doctoral theses, been a peer reviewer for a wide range of journals and several competitive research schemes in Australia and elsewhere, as well as assessing paramedicine education programmes locally and internationally. A highlight of his research has been the opportunity to work collaboratively with doctoral candidates and a wide range of researchers across the globe. The main foci of his recent research have been the evolution of paramedicine as a health discipline, community paramedicine, and the challenge of better understanding the rise in violence perpetrated against paramedics and other health workers.

Walter Tavares, PhD
Walter is a distinguished university professor based in Canada, with a strong focus on advancing health professions education and professional practice, specifically within paramedicine.

He is an Assistant Professor in the Department of Health and Society, Director of the Paramedicine Collaborative in the Department of Family and Community Medicine, and Education Scientist in the Wilson Centre for Health Professions Education Research at the University of Toronto. He is also a Co-Chair of the McNally Project for Paramedicine Research and leads a Research and Development programme with York Region Paramedic Services in Ontario, Canada. He is also a Deputy Editor of the journal *Paramedicine*. He completed his PhD in Health Services Research and a five-year education fellowship at the Wilson Centre. As an experienced academic, Walter's research contributes to educational advances, refinements to clinical and professional practice, and policy development locally, nationally, and internationally. Walter's contributions extend beyond academia into policy advocacy, ensuring advances to evolving challenges.

Julia Williams, PhD
Julia is a registered paramedic who is a Professor of Paramedic Science at the University of Hertfordshire where she has been involved in pre- and post-registration education and development for paramedics since 1996. In addition, as the Head of Research for the College of Paramedics, Julia is committed to increasing the capacity and capability of paramedics within paramedic research, and she takes every opportunity to inform other agencies about the rich talent that exists within the paramedic profession in relation to clinical research, highlighting the positive contribution paramedics make to the health and care research agenda. Over the years, she has gained extensive experience in qualitative, quantitative, and mixed methods research studies related to different aspects of paramedic practice; unscheduled emergency and urgent healthcare provision; paramedic education; and the health and well-being of the paramedic workforce including a national study during the COVID-19 pandemic. She continues to lead research in the South East Coast Ambulance Service NHS Foundation Trust and is an active member of the National Ambulance Research Steering Group (NARSG). Over the years, Julia has sat on several trial steering groups and has been involved in a variety of funding panels and

committees. Amongst other activities, she is an Editor-in-Chief for the *British Paramedic Journal* and a previous Deputy Editor for *Paramedicine*, and she has had the privilege of mentoring several paramedic PhD students during their initial research journeys.

About the Editors

Gregory Adam Whitley, PhD
Greg is an Associate Professor in Paramedic Science at the University of Lincoln and a Paramedic Research Fellow with the East Midlands Ambulance Service NHS Trust. He joined the UK ambulance service in 2010 and became a registered paramedic in 2012.

He completed his PhD in 2020 titled 'Pre-hospital pain management in children: A mixed methods study' and his research interests include the pre-hospital setting and the paramedic profession. He has secured £500k worth of research funding as chief investigator/co-applicant and has helped to deliver research worth over £5m, including the AIRWAYS 2 and PARAMEDIC 3 clinical trials. He has over

40 peer-reviewed publications including empirical research articles, reviews, methodology papers, conference proceedings, and a co-edited textbook titled *Prehospital Research Methods and Practice*. He also has editorial board experience, having served on the *Journal of Paramedic Practice* and the *British Paramedic Journal*.

Greg was awarded a prestigious Advanced Clinical and Practitioner Academic Fellowship in 2023, making him the first paramedic in England to receive a Health Education England/National Institute for Health and Care Research-funded postdoctoral fellowship. The fellowship will fund a programme of research aiming to develop and test an intervention to improve pre-hospital acute pain management for children and young people.

Scott Fraser Sim Munro, PhD

Scott is a Clinical Academic splitting his time equally between clinical practice as a Specialist Paramedic in critical care for the South East Coast Ambulance Service NHS Trust, based in Surrey in South East England, and as a Lecturer in paramedic practice at the University of Surrey, School of Health Sciences. Scott qualified as a paramedic in 2012 and has been working as a Specialist Paramedic since 2019. In 2020, he completed his PhD, which was a mixed method study into the pre-hospital care of acute stroke patients. He co-authored the UK Joint Royal Colleges Ambulance Liaison Committee (JRCALC) clinical stroke guidelines. He has published and presented on several different facets of pre-hospital care both nationally and internationally. His research interests include improving pre-hospital clinical care, improving staff well-being, and the implementation of innovative technologies. He is passionate about bridging research and practice and empowering paramedics to engage in research, emphasising its impact beyond academia as a vital tool for advancing real-world patient care.

List of Case Study Authors

	Name	Job Title	Country
Case Studies—Novice Researchers	Hannah Lindsay	Ambulance Paramedic	Australia
	Alex Diffley	Research Paramedic	United Kingdom
	Owen Stanley	Research Paramedic	United Kingdom
	Andrew Cole	Lead Research Paramedic	United Kingdom
Case Studies—Competent Researchers	Alanowd Alghaith	Teaching Assistant and PhD Student	Saudi Arabia and United Kingdom
	Cheryl Cameron	Director of Operations, PhD Candidate, and Senior Fellow	Canada and Australia
	Thomas Hofmann	Paramedic and Lecturer	Germany
	Ryan Matthews	Lecturer and PhD Candidate	South Africa
Case Studies—Proficient Researchers	Dr Kathryn Eastwood	Associate Professor and Intensive Care Paramedic	Australia
	Dr Caitlin Wilson	Senior Research Fellow (Paramedic)	United Kingdom
	Dr Graham McClelland	Vice Chancellors' Fellow and Honorary Research Fellow, Visiting Clinical Researcher, and Visiting Professor	United Kingdom
Case Studies—Expert Researchers	Dr Willem Stassen	Associate Professor	South Africa
	Professor William (Bill) Lord AM	Adjunct Professor	Australia
	Professor Brian Maguire	Senior Epidemiologist and Adjunct Professor	United States and Australia
	Professor Nigel Rees QAM	Assistant Director of Research, Innovation, and Visiting Professor	United Kingdom

Foreword

I wholeheartedly commend this textbook with a full heart, as it captures the vital, transformative journey of paramedic clinical academics and researchers, celebrating their impact and their boundless potential. This work shines a light on a community that not only lives and breathes in the lives of paramedics but also in the lives of the patients they serve, championing both advocacy and innovation in equal measure.

It is impossible to overstate the importance of the pioneers who have laid the foundation for paramedic research. Professor Malcolm Woollard's contribution from the College of Paramedics' perspective stands as an enduring example of the brilliance and dedication that inspires us all—his contributions continue to resonate as a beacon of possibility for current and future paramedics pursuing research careers, along with an army of others.

The stories, case studies, and achievements chronicled in this textbook are a testament to the evolution and continual improvement of the paramedic profession. They demonstrate how problem-solving and ingenuity are unleashing our potential, positioning paramedics as patient and profession advocates, credible future leaders, and role models. Clinical academics bridge the gap between research and practice, ensuring that studies are relevant to real-world challenges. These dual roles help align research questions with the practical needs of patients and healthcare systems. The research landscape is not without its challenges, and gratitude is owed to those who, despite the hurdles, persevere in advancing the profession with unwavering commitment and tenacity.

Research provides more than knowledge alone—it equips individuals with an unparalleled range of transferable skills, including leadership, strategic thinking, and the agency to enact meaningful change. Supporting employed paramedics in realising their research aspirations is not a luxury but an urgent necessity. Providing opportunities for clinicians to engage in research helps retain skilled professionals in academia, ensuring a continuous flow of expertise and the development of future clinical researchers. This is not the time to be short-sighted. Instead, we must embrace a vision that values diverse perspectives and fosters a research community where shared understanding is pivotal and is one that can create meaningful change.

Paramedic researchers are often disruptors and innovators, challenging the status quo and creating new paradigms of care. This spirit of ingenuity is not merely desirable, it is essential for shaping the future of healthcare. I celebrate and support those who are carving this path and welcome their contributions to a field that continues to redefine itself through bold ambition and unyielding curiosity—something the profession itself has in abundance.

For me, this textbook is more than a collection of insights. It is a call to action for the entire profession to champion the importance of research in unleashing the full potential of paramedics. It is with great pride and renewed optimism that I commend this remarkable work to all who read it.

Tracy Nicholls, OBE FCPara
Chief Executive
College of Paramedics

Preface

We are excited to introduce this novel textbook, the first to provide professional practice development guidance and case study exemplars for paramedics who wish to focus their career on research. Whilst all paramedics pursue careers that involve varying proportions of clinical practice, education, leadership, and research, this textbook is aimed at those wishing to focus a significant proportion of their career on research activities.

The idea for the textbook stemmed, in part, from the online international *Paramedic PhD* registry, which was developed by Greg Whitley in November 2017. The registry accepts voluntary submissions of doctoral-level qualification details in the field of paramedicine internationally.

As of February 2025, 305 doctorates have been registered, of which 268 were from paramedics around the globe. The idea for the registry was conceived by Scott Munro and Tom Quinn during a conversation on Twitter (now X) in 2017 about paramedics who were studying for or had completed a PhD:

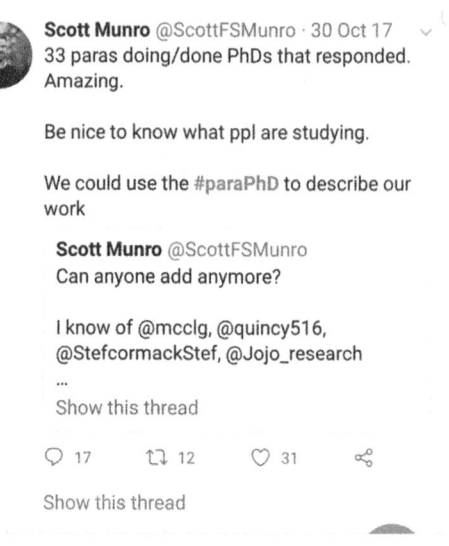

When designing the textbook, we wanted to provide a 'real-world' perspective of what it is like for a paramedic to navigate a career focused on research. From our own personal experience, and that shared by colleagues nationally and internationally, it was clear that there was no single pathway to pursue research. Some jump from Bachelor's degree to Doctoral-level education, some focus on research delivery, others self-fund their education, and some simply step into and out of research at multiple points during their career. To articulate this diversity in approach and provide this 'real-world' perspective, we felt it best to provide case studies from paramedics across the globe at various stages of their career.

We then wanted to define the stages of a paramedic career that focused on research. This was harder than we thought. Building on the work of the Dreyfus brothers in 1980, Benner [1] proposed five stages of proficiency in 1982: Novice, Advanced Beginner, Competent, Proficient, and Expert. We used this as an underlying framework and mapped out what we felt were key research activities, such as participation, delivery, design, funding acquisition, and leadership. We also considered, to a somewhat greater degree of difficulty, the education levels paramedics might undertake and achieve at the different stages. We soon realised this was much more fluid and was not amenable to simple categorisation. Therefore, we loosely associated the educational level to each career stage, rather than being prescriptive (many notable professors do not have a PhD, for example, and some who do have a PhD may undertake limited research activities). With all this consideration, we felt five stages were too many, so the Advanced Beginner stage was removed to leave a four-stage model. The final decision for the model was to illustrate that as one progresses through the career stages, research activities that are lower down in the model are still undertaken at the higher stages, even when reaching senior career positions such as Consultant, Director, or Professor; therefore, a pyramid structure was deemed appropriate to capture this progressive and inclusive nature. For example, a professor may still participate in research and complete a survey or be interviewed. The final paramedic research career stage model can be found in **Chapter 1—Figure 1.1.**

We were keen to source expert contributors for the text-book, by both knowledge and experience. **Section 1** provides the overview and background context relating to the history of the ambulance service, the paramedic profession, and paramedics in academia, along with consideration for education when navigating a research career. Scott and Greg provide the introduction in Chapter 1, both UK postdoctoral registered paramedics focusing their careers on research. With his vast clinical experience and recent co-authored editorial titled 'The Evolution of Clinician-Academics in Paramedicine: Completing the Picture of Professionalism' [2], Ben Meadley was well suited to author Chapter 2. With experience in the paramedic education systems at an international level across Ireland, Canada, and Australia, Alan Batt along with Brendan Shannon, who is an experienced leader in curriculum development in Australia, were both well suited to co-author Chapter 3.

Section 2 explores the four-stage career model, providing case studies for each and a discussion of the benefits and challenges at each level. It was important that each chapter author in this section was an expert by experience, therefore, we recruited who we considered to either be at or towards the end of each respective career stage. This enabled the chapter authors to blend excerpts from the case studies for each chapter and also inject their own experience and knowledge, creating truly exceptional 'real-world' chapters. Elisha Miller (United Kingdom), Georgette Eaton (United Kingdom), Walter Tavares (Canada), and Peter O'Meara and Malcolm Boyle (Australia) have authored Chapters 4, 5, 6, and 7, respectively.

Section 3 provides expert advice from the longest-standing Professor of Paramedic Science in the United

Kingdom, the Head of Research in the College of Paramedics, and the Head of Research for South East Coast Ambulance Service in the United Kingdom, Julia Williams. Julia provides a question-and-answer style chapter, composed of a multitude of questions posed to Julia over the years regarding research in paramedic practice.

We would like to take this opportunity to sincerely thank all the chapter authors involved in drafting this important resource, the contributing case study authors for providing their 'real-world' insights, and the peer reviewers for their extremely valuable contribution to this textbook. We would like to thank Caitlin Wilson for critically reviewing aspects of the textbook. We would also like to thank Tracy Nicholls for providing the Foreword.

As a collective effort, we have created something truly special.

Greg and Scott.

References

1. Benner, P. (1982). From novice to expert. *The American Journal of Nursing* 82 (3): 402–407.
2. Meadley, B.N., Andrews, T., Delardes, B.J., and Shannon, B.P. (2022). The evolution of clinician–academics in paramedicine: completing the picture of professionalism. *Prehospital and Disaster Medicine* 37 (5): 574–576.

Section 1

Setting the Scene for Clinical Academic Paramedics

Chapter 1

The Role and Importance of Clinical Academics in Paramedicine

Scott Fraser Sim Munro[1,2] and Gregory Adam Whitley[3,4]

[1] School of Health Sciences, University of Surrey, Guildford, United Kingdom

[2] Nexus House, South East Coast Ambulance Service NHS Trust, Crawley, United Kingdom

[3] School of Health and Care Sciences, University of Lincoln, Lincoln, United Kingdom

[4] Clinical Audit and Research Unit, East Midlands Ambulance Service NHS Trust, Lincoln, United Kingdom

Research-focused Careers for Paramedics, First Edition.
Edited by Gregory A. Whitley and Scott Munro.
© 2025 John Wiley & Sons Ltd. Published 2025 by John Wiley & Sons Ltd.

Chapter Objectives

1. Introduce the role and importance of clinical academics in paramedicine.
2. Define clinical academic responsibilities and the value of research.
3. Highlight benefits of a research career.
4. Address barriers and strategies to overcome them.
5. Outline funding options for aspiring clinical academics.

What Is a Clinical Academic?

The intersection of clinical practice and research is where true innovation in healthcare occurs. Clinical academics are at the forefront of this intersection, blending the roles of healthcare provider and researcher, which enables them to deliver high-quality evidence-based education. This chapter explores the important role of clinical academics within the paramedic profession, highlighting how their unique blend of skills and experiences drives advancements in patient care and healthcare knowledge.

Clinical academics are healthcare professionals who combine clinical practice with research and often teaching. They split their time between providing patient care, conducting research, and training the next generation of clinicians, typically working across healthcare systems and universities. Some clinical academics choose to split their time 50:50 across clinical and research roles, while others choose different ratios that may fluctuate over time depending on research, teaching, and clinical demands. The nature of clinical academic work is diverse, shaped by their specialism, experience, interests, and the specific demands of the healthcare and academic environments in which they operate.

Paramedics, with their firsthand experience of healthcare challenges, are uniquely positioned to conduct research that directly impacts patient care. Whilst the profession is relatively new (discussed further in **Chapter 2**), it has made significant advances in a relatively short period of time. They understand the most pressing issues in the systems they work in and can identify practical solutions that improve outcomes. This *insider knowledge* allows them to design research that is not only relevant but also highly impactful, addressing gaps that might be overlooked by those outside the profession.

The role of a clinical academic is thus multifaceted. By bringing the benefits of high-quality research directly to patient care, they help contribute to improved outcomes through evidence-based practices. Their involvement in academia allows them to add significantly to the scientific community, fostering advancements in healthcare knowledge and practice.

Terminology

We use the term 'clinical academic' throughout this chapter to describe the career of a paramedic who maintains their role in clinical practice *and* undertakes research activities. However, we understand this term does not suit all, and many senior paramedic researchers and educators no longer work in clinical practice.

(continued)

> *(continued)*
>
> Other terms may be more appropriate here, such as 'practitioner academic' or 'pracademic'. We have chosen to use the term 'clinical academic' due to its ubiquity in international literature.

The Importance and Benefits of Clinical Academic Careers

Engaging in research is vital for paramedics, as it plays a crucial role in advancing patient care, enhancing professional development, and improving healthcare organisations. Paramedics, with their firsthand experience of the challenges in emergency medical services, are uniquely positioned to conduct research that directly addresses these issues, leading to practical and impactful solutions.

Benefits to the Individual

For paramedics, pursuing a career that includes research offers many personal and professional benefits. On a personal level, research provides intellectual stimulation and the satisfaction of contributing to the advancement of knowledge in their profession [1]. It encourages continuous learning, endless curiosity, critical thinking and pushes you to delve deeper into your areas of interest and develop new expertise.

Professionally, engaging in research enhances critical thinking, problem-solving, and data analysis skills—competencies that are essential for effective clinical practice. These skills contribute to better decision-making and ultimately improve patient care. Additionally, research activities open doors to professional recognition and career advancement. Paramedics involved in research have opportunities to publish their findings, present at conferences, and collaborate with other experts, thereby establishing themselves as leaders in their field.

Furthermore, research can lead to further educational opportunities, such as advanced degrees or specialised training programs (discussed further in **Chapter 3**). These qualifications not only enhance the paramedic's knowledge and skills but also improve their career prospects and potential for leadership roles within their organisations.

Benefits to Patients

One of the primary goals of research is to improve patient outcomes through evidence-based practice. Research conducted by paramedics is directly informed by their frontline experiences and can result in the development of innovative care strategies. This ensures that new treatments and interventions are both practical and effective.

Research allows for the identification and implementation of best practices in patient care. This leads to more effective and efficient treatment protocols, reducing the risk of errors and improving overall patient safety. By staying at the forefront of medical advancements, paramedics can provide the highest quality of care to their patients [2].

Benefits to Organisations

Supporting clinical research within health and care organisations offers numerous advantages. Research-active environments are known for delivering superior patient care, as clinical academics foster a culture of continuous improvement and evidence-based practice [2, 3]. This ensures that clinical guidelines and protocols are consistently updated with the latest research, leading to better patient outcomes and enhanced trust in healthcare services.

Integrating research into practice also boosts organisational efficiency. By applying research findings, organisations can streamline processes, reduce inefficiencies, and make better use of resources. This not only leads to cost savings but also optimises service delivery, ensuring that patients receive the best possible care. Additionally, successful research initiatives can attract grant funding and other financial resources, further supporting the organisation's goals.

Clinical academics bring advanced analytical and problem-solving skills to the organisation, promoting a more rigorous and data-driven approach to healthcare delivery. Their expertise in research methodologies contributes to a deeper understanding of complex issues, resulting in improved care quality and organisational performance.

Organisations that prioritise research are more likely to attract and retain high-calibre staff. The opportunity to engage in meaningful research can foster a rewarding work environment that enhances job satisfaction and professional development. This focus on research can also lead to a happier, more fulfilled workforce, reducing burnout and improving overall staff well-being [4].

Finally, having clinical academics on board signals a commitment to excellence and innovation, enhancing the organisation's reputation within the healthcare community. This can lead to increased opportunities for collaboration with other institutions and industry partners, further advancing the organisation's mission and impact.

Introducing the Clinical Academic Pathway

Building a clinical academic career is an incremental and sometimes challenging process, but it can also be extremely rewarding and essential for the progression of the paramedic profession. This book provides clear guidance and support by structuring content around the stages of this pathway, visualised in the accompanying model (**Figure 1.1**). While every researcher's journey is unique, with individuals joining, progressing, and sometimes exiting at different points, this model offers a helpful framework to make sense of the varied paths one might take. The pathway outlines the progression from novice to expert researcher, highlighting key leadership roles and responsibilities at each stage. These stages not only serve as a roadmap for paramedics, offering a clear route for career development and professional growth, but also form the structure of the rest of the book itself.

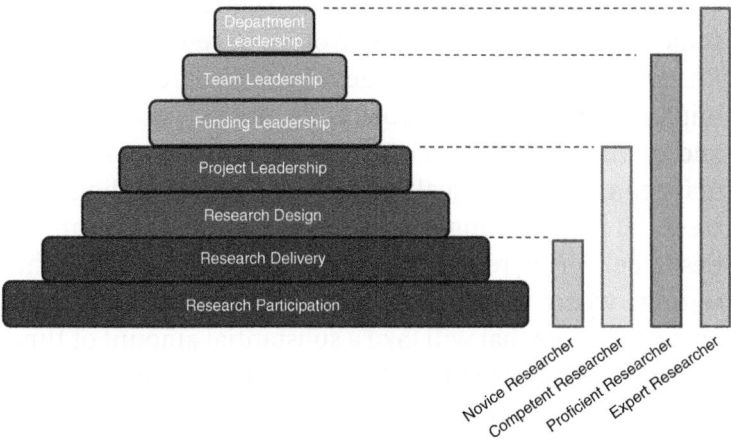

Figure 1.1 Clinical Academic Career Model

Each chapter corresponds to a different level of researcher, allowing readers to follow the journey from novice to expert, understanding the specific challenges and opportunities at each stage.

Stages of the Clinical Academic Pathway

Novice Researcher

The journey of a clinical academic begins at the novice stage, where the focus is on building a strong foundation in research. Novice researchers are introduced to the basic elements of research, gaining hands-on experience that is crucial for their future roles.

Research Participation: Novice researchers gain foundational knowledge and experience by engaging in research projects. They participate in tasks such as completing surveys, taking part in interviews, and recruiting participants. This stage emphasises hands-on experience and understanding the basic processes involved in research.

Research Delivery: At this stage, novice researchers assist in implementing research projects, including data collection and preliminary analysis. They learn the basics of project management and ethical research practices, building skills essential for executing research plans. Given the complexities of delivering research in ambulance services and other settings where paramedics work, research delivery is an area of practice that will take a substantial amount of time, skill, and experience to master. A career in research delivery can be both satisfying and valid in itself—some paramedics may have no desire or need to progress any further along the proposed clinical academic career model. See **Chapter 4** for case studies and further exploration of the Novice Researcher career stage.

Competent Researcher

As some researchers progress to the competent stage, they begin to take on more responsibility and leadership within research projects. This phase marks the transition from participant to leader, with a focus on research design and project management.

Research Design: In addition to previous responsibilities, competent researchers design research projects, develop protocols, and formulate research questions. This stage requires a comprehensive understanding of research design principles and the ability to critically evaluate existing literature.

Project Leadership: Competent researchers take on leadership roles, overseeing research projects from planning to completion. They coordinate team activities, manage timelines, and ensure project goals are met, fostering a collaborative environment. See **Chapter 5** for case studies and more details of the Competent Researcher career stage.

Proficient Researcher

At the proficient stage, researchers have developed significant expertise and are entrusted with leading teams and securing funding for their projects. This stage is characterised by a deep engagement with research and the broader academic community.

Funding Leadership: At this stage, researchers lead efforts to secure funding, often acting as lead applicants on grant proposals. They manage the financial aspects of research, from writing successful grant applications to maintaining budget oversight, which is critical for sustaining research initiatives.

Team Leadership: Proficient researchers lead research teams, managing research assistants, fellows, principal investigators, patient and public involvement groups, along with other key stakeholder groups, and work closely with core members of the research team. They are responsible for the strategic direction of projects, ensuring high-quality outputs, and mentoring junior team members. See **Chapter 6** for case studies and discussion of the Proficient Researcher career stage.

Expert Researcher

The expert stage represents the pinnacle of a clinical academic career, where researchers take on significant leadership roles within their organisations. They influence research agendas at the departmental level and play a key role in shaping healthcare policy and strategy.

Department Leadership: Expert researchers take on leadership roles at the departmental level, directing research and shaping agendas. They influence broader research policy and strategy, representing their department in academic and professional forums. This stage involves significant responsibilities, including administrative duties, policy development, and advocacy within the healthcare and education systems. See **Chapter 7** for case studies and an exploration of the Expert Researcher career stage.

Challenges and Barriers to Becoming a Clinical Academic

While the benefits of becoming a clinical academic are substantial, there are also significant barriers that can deter paramedics from pursuing this career path. A primary challenge lies in the lack of awareness and understanding of the clinical academic pathway within the paramedic profession. Many paramedics are simply unaware of the opportunities available, leading to underutilisation of this career option. This lack of awareness is compounded by limited access to research training and mentorship, making it difficult for paramedics to acquire the necessary skills and guidance to embark on a research-focused career [5]. The concept of *"you can't be what you can't see"* [Marian Wright Edelman] also poses a challenge here, due to the lack of role models within the paramedic profession, as so few have currently reached the expert stage.

Securing adequate funding and resources presents another major hurdle. Research roles often depend on competitive grants, which can lead to financial instability for those transitioning into academic positions. The insecurity of fixed-term contracts within research represents a significant challenge for paramedics wishing to pursue research-orientated roles. The pressure to secure funding, coupled with the challenge of balancing clinical duties with research commitments, can result in an increased workload and heightened stress, contributing to the risk of burnout. The transition from clinical to academic roles also introduces career uncertainty, as paramedics navigate new responsibilities and expectations. However, while these challenges are daunting, they are not insurmountable [5].

Overcoming Barriers and Addressing Challenges

Overcoming these barriers requires a concerted effort from both individuals and the wider healthcare and academic systems. For paramedics aspiring to become clinical academics, enhancing their understanding about the clinical academic pathway is a crucial first step. Targeted outreach and education initiatives by institutions and professional organisations can play a significant role in promoting the benefits and opportunities of research-focused careers, encouraging more paramedics to explore this path. However, increasing visibility alone is not enough. Without the active cooperation and support of institutions in providing the necessary time, resources, and funding, these career pathways remain inaccessible for many.

Securing institutional support and funding is another critical area where both individual initiative and systemic change are needed. While paramedics can work on developing strong research proposals and building a network of collaborators to increase their chances of securing funding, it is also important for healthcare institutions and universities to advocate for increased funding and institutional support. Joint appointments between healthcare institutions and higher education establishments may provide a stable foundation for balancing clinical and academic responsibilities, allowing clinical academics to thrive in both environments.

A key element in overcoming these barriers is the mentorship and guidance provided by experienced paramedic researchers, along with other experienced healthcare researchers and methodologists. It is important for aspiring clinical academic paramedics to seek mentorship and formal supervision not only from experienced paramedic researchers but also from others who have *topic, population, setting,* or *methodological* expertise. For example, when pursuing research focused on children and young people, it would be wise to seek mentorship or supervision from a paediatrician, or a Professor of Child Health, for example. Similarly, when undertaking a research project that involves statistical analysis, it would be wise to seek mentorship or supervision from a medical statistician. Hence, networking and collaboration are key. The next generation of clinical academics can greatly benefit from the wisdom and experience of those who have already navigated the complexities of a research career. Experienced researchers can offer invaluable insights, helping to build the confidence and competence required for success. By actively mentoring and supporting emerging researchers, these seasoned professionals play a crucial role in sustaining and expanding the clinical academic community within paramedicine.

Access to research training and mentorship is vital for building the skills necessary for a successful research career. Individuals can seek out mentors and take advantage of available training programmes to develop their research abilities. However, it is also essential for institutions to expand these opportunities, ensuring that aspiring researchers have the support they need to navigate the complexities of research. Experienced academics can guide trainees through the research process, helping them to build a solid foundation for their careers.

Building a supportive network is equally important for overcoming the challenges of a clinical academic career. By connecting with peers and joining professional communities, paramedics can share knowledge and experiences, building resilience and fostering continued growth throughout their careers. Institutions can facilitate this by creating platforms for collaboration and peer support, ensuring that clinical academics do not face these challenges in isolation. Effective career planning is another key factor in overcoming barriers. Paramedics considering a research career should communicate early with their clinical service managers, providing advance notice of their intentions. This allows managers to plan for backfilling positions and make a case for releasing paramedics' time for research. Incorporating research training plans into personal development plans can also help to formalise the career trajectory and ensure that both clinical and academic goals are aligned.

Flexibility in research focus is important for sustained professional development. While integrating research expertise into the clinician's current service can be a practical starting point, it is crucial to maintain the flexibility to explore different research areas as the career progresses. This adaptability allows clinical academics to respond to emerging trends and challenges in their field, ensuring that their research remains relevant and impactful.

Aligning research projects with organisational goals is another strategy that can help to secure support and resources. By understanding the challenges and priorities of managers and organisations, paramedics can design research that contributes to quality improvement initiatives and enhances patient care, management, and overall healthcare services.

Finally, promoting diversity within clinical academia is essential for creating an inclusive environment for all researchers. Peer support and mentorship are particularly vital for underrepresented groups, who may face additional and unique challenges in accessing opportunities and advancing their careers. Increasing diversity within clinical academia strengthens the academic community, fostering inclusivity and enhancing the relevance and impact of our research by ensuring that we conduct research reflective of the diverse populations we serve for equitable care and meaningful findings.

By addressing these challenges head-on, through both individual efforts and systemic changes, paramedics can overcome the barriers to becoming successful clinical academics and make a significant impact on their profession. The combined efforts of individuals and institutions are essential to creating an environment where clinical academics can thrive, ultimately benefiting the entire healthcare system.

The following chapters, along with the included case studies and insights from contributing authors, provide further advice and guidance on navigating some of the hurdles of a paramedic clinical academic career. These resources are designed to offer practical strategies, inspiration, and support as you embark on or continue your journey in this vital and rewarding field. The final chapter (**Chapter 8**) offers expert advice on clinical academic career progression.

Funding Options

Securing funding is a critical aspect of building a successful career as a clinical academic. Without adequate financial support, research activities cannot be sustained, access to necessary resources is limited, and financial stability becomes uncertain. Funding is, therefore, the backbone of a thriving research career, enabling researchers to pursue their academic goals and contribute to advancements in healthcare. However, securing funding can be one of the most challenging aspects of establishing a clinical academic career.

Navigating the Funding Landscape

Aspiring clinical academics have a range of funding options at their disposal, including government grants, academic scholarships, fellowships, support from professional organisations and charitable foundations, and industry partnerships. Each pathway offers unique opportunities and challenges, and researchers often forge their own unique paths by combining these and other sources of funding.

Securing funding is often a highly competitive process, requiring researchers to submit detailed proposals that clearly outline the potential impact and significance of their work. Crafting these grant applications is a time-consuming and demanding task, and initial applications are not always successful. However, setbacks should not discourage researchers completely. Even though it may initially feel redundant, feedback from reviewers can provide valuable insights that help refine and improve projects for future submissions. Sometimes, it may be necessary to recognise when a project has reached its natural conclusion and shift focus to new ideas. Collaborating with experienced academics during this process can provide crucial support and guidance, helping to navigate the challenges of securing funding. It's important to remember that rejection is a normal part of the research journey and something almost all researchers will experience at some point. It's not a reflection of your personal worth or abilities. Instead, consider it a stepping stone in your growth as a researcher—an opportunity to learn, refine your ideas, and come back stronger.

Government Grants, Fellowships, and Research Funding Programs

Government grants are often the cornerstone of funding for clinical academics. These grants, typically offered by national funding bodies, are designed to support research that aligns with public health priorities. They offer a variety of grants for different stages of research, from initial project development to large-scale, complex clinical trials. These grants are crucial for addressing key health challenges and ensuring that funded research has a significant impact on public health. Government bodies may also fund fellowships—personal training awards that focus on training and development, whilst also undertaking a program of research.

Academic Institution Scholarships and Fellowships

Academic institutions frequently offer scholarships and fellowships to support clinical academics, particularly those in the early stages of their careers. These awards can cover a range of needs, including salaries, research expenses, travel, and conference attendance, offering comprehensive support for academic growth.

Many universities and colleges have institution-specific programmes tailored to nurture their academic community. These scholarships and fellowships are invaluable for budding researchers, providing the resources and opportunities needed to advance their careers. Early-career researchers should actively explore these options and consider how they align with their long-term goals.

Many scholarships and fellowships fund postgraduate masters and doctoral-level study and are often considered career development awards (rather than research grants) as they facilitate the transition of clinical academics from one stage to the next.

Professional Organisations and Charitable Foundations

Professional organisations and foundations play a significant role in funding research, particularly within specific fields of study. These entities often focus on advancing particular areas of knowledge and supporting researchers dedicated to those fields. Grants and fellowships from professional organisations and charitable foundations are typically aimed at funding innovative research projects and supporting early-career researchers.

In addition to financial support, these organisations often provide mentorship opportunities and networking events, helping researchers build connections and advance their careers. Securing funding from these sources can be competitive, requiring a strong demonstration of the project's relevance and potential impact. Nonetheless, these grants are invaluable for researchers aiming to make significant contributions to their fields.

Research Grants versus Fellowships

The choice between applying for a research grant versus a fellowship is a personal one. There is no right or wrong answer here, but they are tailored to slightly different needs. If you are looking for an award with more support and training, then you may consider personal awards and fellowships. If you are confident in your research ability and have a strong research team, you may consider research grants. Some may apply for both.

Industry Partnerships and Collaborations

Collaborations with industry partners can be a valuable source of funding and support for clinical academics. These partnerships often involve working with pharmaceutical companies, medical device manufacturers, and other healthcare-related businesses. Industry partners may fund joint research projects that align with their strategic interests, providing access to additional resources and expertise.

Sponsored research agreements, a common form of industry collaboration, involve funding-specific research activities at academic institutions. These agreements often include provisions for intellectual property sharing and publication rights. Industry partnerships can also offer internships and secondments, allowing researchers to gain practical experience and apply their academic knowledge in real-world settings.

Securing industry funding requires careful negotiation and alignment of research goals with industry interests. While challenging, these collaborations can provide substantial support and open new avenues for research and development. Researchers should approach these partnerships with a clear understanding of mutual goals and potential benefits.

Exploring Small Grant Schemes

While securing large grants can be a cornerstone of funding a significant research project, it is equally important to be aware of smaller grant schemes that many organisations offer. These small grants may not fully cover the costs of extensive research projects, but they can be incredibly valuable for providing financial support for smaller initiatives or for researchers who are just starting out.

Small grants often serve as a stepping stone, enabling researchers to undertake pilot studies, gather preliminary data, or explore innovative ideas on a smaller scale. These projects can be crucial for building a track record of successful research, which in turn strengthens future applications for larger grants.

Organisations such as professional associations, foundations, and even some universities frequently offer these small grant opportunities. While the funding amounts may be modest, they can still cover essential expenses such as travel, equipment, or participant incentives, helping to move your research forward. Additionally, these smaller grants often come with fewer strings attached and a more streamlined application process, making them more accessible to early-career researchers. They can also provide a great opportunity to gain experience in grant writing and management without the pressure of handling large-scale funding.

For those new to research, these small grants can be an excellent way to start building your portfolio and gaining the confidence needed to tackle more substantial projects in the future. Keep an eye out for these opportunities, as they can make a significant difference in getting your research off the ground.

The Challenges of Contract-Based Employment

Many clinical academic careers are built on a series of fixed-term contracts, a common arrangement in higher education and research fields. While these contracts can offer flexibility and opportunities for diverse experiences, they also come with challenges.

The temporary nature of these positions can lead to job insecurity, as researchers are constantly evaluated on their performance, and employment can be terminated relatively easily. This insecurity can create stress and uncertainty, making it difficult to plan long-term career paths or personal lives.

On the other hand, some individuals appreciate the flexibility that contract-based employment offers. These roles may allow researchers to explore external opportunities and construct their own professional identities. Moving between different projects and institutions can lead to a varied career, fostering a wide range of skills and experiences.

Ultimately, securing funding and managing a clinical academic career require strategic planning and resilience. Researchers must be proactive in exploring various funding sources, continuously refining their proposals, and building strong networks of collaborators and mentors. Institutions, in turn, must advocate for increased funding and provide the necessary support structures to help clinical academics thrive.

As you navigate these challenges, remember that the journey of securing funding is as much about persistence and adaptation as it is about skill and knowledge. We hope that the insights and strategies outlined in this book will help you forge a successful and fulfilling career as a clinical academic, making meaningful contributions to both your field and the broader healthcare landscape.

Chapter Summary

In summary, the journey of a clinical academic in the paramedic profession is both challenging and deeply rewarding. This chapter has provided you with a roadmap for navigating the various stages of this career path, from the initial steps of securing funding and mentorship to the long-term challenges of balancing clinical and academic responsibilities. The insights shared here are intended to equip you with the knowledge and strategies needed to overcome obstacles and seize opportunities as they arise.

As you reflect on the content of this chapter, remember that your path will be unique, shaped by your experiences, interests, and goals. While the barriers may seem daunting, they are not insurmountable. With determination, support, and a strategic approach, you can build a successful clinical academic career that not only advances your own professional development but also contributes to the growth and improvement of the paramedic profession as a whole.

The following chapters will delve deeper into specific aspects of this journey, offering case studies, expert advice, and practical tools to further guide you. We hope that the knowledge and guidance provided in this book will serve as a strong foundation as you continue to pursue your ambitions in clinical academia.

References

1. Whitley, G.A. and Wilson, C. (2022). Paramedics ... Why do research? *British Paramedic Journal* 7 (1): 1–2.
2. Boaz, A., Hanney, S., Jones, T., and Soper, B. (2015). Does the engagement of clinicians and organisations in research improve healthcare performance: a three-stage review. *BMJ Open* 5 (12): e009415.

3. Chalmers, S., Hill, J., Connell, L. et al. (2023). The value of allied health professional research engagement on healthcare performance: a systematic review. *BMC Health Services Research* 23 (1): 766.

4. Zhuang, C., Hu, X., and Dill, M.J. (2022). Do physicians with academic affiliation have lower burnout and higher career-related satisfaction? *BMC Medical Education* 22 (1): 316.

5. Trusson, D., Rowley, E., and Bramley, L. (2019). A mixed-methods study of challenges and benefits of clinical academic careers for nurses, midwives and allied health professionals. *BMJ Open* 9 (10): e030595.

Chapter 2

History of Ambulance Services, Paramedics, and Research in Paramedicine

Ben Meadley

Department of Paramedicine, Monash University, Melbourne, Victoria, Australia

Research-focused Careers for Paramedics, First Edition.
Edited by Gregory A. Whitley and Scott Munro.
© 2025 John Wiley & Sons Ltd. Published 2025 by John Wiley & Sons Ltd.

Chapter Objectives

1. Provide a historical overview of the ambulance service from an international perspective.
2. Describe the progression of the paramedic profession.
3. Discuss the transition of paramedics into research and academia.

Introduction

Paramedicine, as a field, has evolved significantly over the last century, and exponentially so in the past three decades. The history of ambulance services and paramedicine more broadly highlights a shift from a primarily skill- and practice-based, trade-like vocation to a profession increasingly grounded in evidence-based practice. This transformation has been driven by the efforts of leaders, paramedics, academics, researchers, and clinician–academics dedicated to improving out-of-hospital care through systematic inquiry and evidence generation. The evolution of paramedicine reflects diverse regional needs, from the development of sophisticated trauma response systems in urban centres to adaptable, community-based models in rural and resource-limited areas across the world.

Early Beginnings and Challenges in Ambulance Services

The origins of organised ambulance services have roots that span continents, evolving in response to military, public health, and social needs. Whilst immediate care principles date back to the Knights Hospitaller of the 12th and 13th centuries [1], the origins of organised ambulance services arose in the late 18th century during the French Revolutionary Wars. Napoleon's medical staff, the *Service de Santé*, recognised the importance of rapid medical response and prompt evacuation from battlefields. The introduction of an ambulance service to the battlefield significantly reduced mortality rates of wounded soldiers through timely medical intervention [2–4].

As is often the case, war provides many lessons, and in the 19th century, civilian ambulance services began to emerge. In 1865, the Commercial Hospital of Cincinnati established the first hospital-based ambulance service in the United States. New York City followed suit with the Bellevue Hospital, which developed the first municipal-based emergency medical services (EMS) system [3, 4]. These early services used horse-drawn carriages and later motorised vehicles to transport patients to hospitals.

In line with increased community engagement with the motor vehicle, the early 20th century saw the expansion of motorised ambulances, improving response times and more timely delivery of unwell patients to hospital. Once more, the inevitability of war led to further advancements in out-of-hospital care. During World Wars I and II, military ambulance services evolved the care of patients suffering traumatic injuries and infectious diseases. The use of stretcher bearers and later medics to provide initial treatment on the battlefield, followed by transportation to field hospitals, laid the groundwork for the modern EMS we know today [2–4]. The Korean and Vietnam Wars further enhanced emergency medical care with the introduction of helicopters, reducing the time from injury to medical care, and the development of major trauma systems of care in the civilian world [5]. The tragedies of more recent wars have greatly enhanced care for those suffering major trauma in civilian communities [6]. The post-war era spawned early educational programs for civilian paramedics. In the 1950s, the basic emergency medical technician (EMT) training program for the Chicago Fire Department laid the foundation for the EMT-Basic certification in the United States that remains today. In 1966, a US National Academy of Sciences paper highlighted out-of-hospital care inadequacies, leading to the creation of the US Department of Transportation's (DOT) National Highway Traffic Safety Administration, which developed standardised EMT training programs. In contrast to the progression of paramedic education into the university sector in the last 25 years, specifically across the United Kingdom and Australasia, the US paramedic system remains linked to these vocational programs, under the auspices of the original US DOT structures [3, 4]. For an example of the evolution of paramedicine in the US, see Box 2.1.

Whilst foundations of out-of-hospital care are well-reported in the United States, the evolution of EMS and paramedic services was parallelled across the developed world. In the United Kingdom, ambulance services have a rich history dating back to the 19th century. The UK's National Health Service (NHS) played a crucial role in organising and improving ambulance services, integrating them into the broader healthcare system [2]. Professor Frank Pantridge pioneered a coronary care ambulance in Belfast in the mid-1960s [7], setting the standard for out-of-hospital critical care and intensive care paramedicine to this day.

In Australia, the St John Ambulance Brigade provided formal ambulance services until the late 1950s, when government-funded ambulance services became more common. The

Australian model innovated with the introduction of mobile intensive care ambulances, staffed with advanced clinicians and doctors [4]. Services akin to Belfast commenced in Melbourne and Sydney, Australia, during the early to mid-1970s, eventually removing the doctor in favour of dual paramedic

Box 2.1
Lessons from History: Freedom House Ambulance Service

A significant chapter in the history of EMS is the Freedom House Ambulance Service, which operated in Pittsburgh, United States, during the late 1960s and early 1970s. This service was a pioneering initiative led by Doctors Peter Safar and Nancy Caroline, aimed at providing high-quality out-of-hospital care while addressing racial and social inequities. Freedom House trained unemployed black citizens from Pittsburgh in the United States, turning them into highly skilled paramedics [8].

The program received international attention for its success in training paramedics and setting standards for emergency medical care. Despite its achievements, Freedom House faced political and financial challenges, ultimately leading to its closure in 1975. However, the program's legacy lived on, influencing EMS systems worldwide.

This example of inclusivity, equity and benevolence led by Dr Nancy Caroline, the author of the seminal paramedic text book 'Emergency Care on the Streets' [9], is a historical example of what is today a modern aspiration.

teams. These systems evolved to form the intensive and critical care paramedic systems we know today. These pioneering systems are the origin of the term paramedic, one that is proudly associated with the noble and respected profession of paramedicine as it is now known.

As well as war, the development of EMS in other regions of the world has often been crisis-driven, shaped by local needs. In Sub-Saharan Africa, for example, EMS systems have been catalysed by public health emergencies, with Sierra Leone establishing its EMS during the 2014–2016 Ebola outbreak. Resources initially deployed for epidemic control were later repurposed for broader emergency care needs, reflecting how localized healthcare challenges influence EMS progression [10].

Evolution of the Paramedic

Paramedic Role

Over the course of more than a century, the paramedic profession has evolved considerably from its origins, where the primary focus was on stretcher-bearers transporting patients directly to hospitals. Early roles like 'ambulance driver', 'ambulance officer', and 'emergency medical technician' were defined by hands-on, technical skills, often drawing individuals from trade or military backgrounds [2, 4]. Today, however, in many settings, paramedics are recognised as registered healthcare professionals with advanced decision-making abilities, playing a vital role in patient care.

Alongside these clinical and patient care advancements, the profession has also gained recognition as part of the broader health sector, aligning with other healthcare roles through registration as healthcare professionals [11, 12]. This transition has been significant in regions such as Australasia, the United Kingdom, the United States, South Africa, and other jurisdictions. This milestone not only enhances patient safety but it also allows the paramedic's role to expand beyond its traditional confines within an ambulance.

Today, paramedics are found in diverse settings: from the traditional ambulance service vehicle to primary healthcare clinics, community outreach programs, hospitals, and academia. These role expansions are closely tied to improved paramedic education and the formal recognition of paramedics as essential healthcare professionals.

Paramedic Education

In various parts of the world—including South Africa, Australia, the United States, and the United Kingdom— paramedic education has evolved significantly over the last 30 years. This transformation has shifted from basic first aid training to comprehensive university degree programs, with each region following its own unique trajectory and achieving distinct milestones.

In the early 1960s, paramedic education in Australia began with the establishment of ambulance service training centres. These centres provided basic training primarily focused on first aid and basic life support. By the late 1970s, the vocational education and training (VET) sector began accrediting education for ambulance officers, marking the start of formalised paramedic education [13, 14]. As previously discussed, in the United States, the need for standardised EMS education was recognised following the 1966 National Academy of Sciences report 'Accidental Death and Disability: The Neglected Disease of Modern Society'. This report highlighted the inadequacies in emergency care and led to the development of formal EMS training programs which remain as primarily vocational programs today [15]. In 1960s England, the 'Millar Report' played a crucial role in shaping paramedic education by specifying training requirements for ambulance personnel. This report led to the introduction of the Ambulance Services Proficiency Certificate, setting the groundwork for future advancements in paramedic training [16]. In Australia, the 1974 Kangan Inquiry into technical education resulted in the establishment of technical and further education (TAFE) as a national entity, providing funding and national standards for vocational training. By the 1980s, paramedic education had advanced to include associate diploma-level training, with states like Victoria and Northern Territory leading the way.

In the United States, the National Highway Traffic Safety Administration (NHTSA) played a pivotal role in advancing and standardising vocational EMS programs. The 1996 'EMS Education Agenda for the Future' proposed a national EMS education system, aiming to amalgamate and advance the training standards across the country [15]. Despite challenges in implementation, this agenda drove quasi-professionalisation of EMS in the United States. At a similar time in the United Kingdom, the Joint Royal Colleges Ambulance Liaison Committee (JRCALC) was established to provide clinical oversight and develop national clinical guidelines, further progressing the professionalisation of paramedics [16].

The move towards university-based education marked a significant shift in paramedic training. Victoria University (Melbourne, Victoria, Australia) and Charles Sturt

University (Bathurst, New South Wales, Australia) were the pioneers of undergraduate paramedic training. These institutions commenced the first paramedic degree conversion programs for employed paramedics in the mid-1990s, beckoning the beginning of the formal transition from vocational programs to higher education [13, 14, 17]. This shift was primarily driven by the need for better academic foundations for advancing clinical skills, increased clinical autonomy, and the drive towards health professional registration.

By the late 1990s, several Australian universities began offering pre-employment paramedic degrees. Jurisdictional ambulance services now had a choice to employ paramedics through a vocational pathway, or already academically qualified with a bachelor's degree. In line with the growth of pre-employment degrees, the Council of Ambulance Authorities (CAA) and other professional bodies developed accreditation standards and competency guidelines to ensure consistent and high-quality education programs [13, 14, 17]. Despite the rigour surrounding degree programs, in early years, cultural barriers remained, limiting the acceptance of the university-trained cohort by vocationally trained paramedics.

In the United States, the transition to higher education has been slower, with community colleges (like TAFE in Australia) primarily offering basic EMT programs. However, some universities have been providing bachelor's degree programs for paramedics, aiming to enhance the level of care and professional status within the field [3, 15]. Whilst national registration is well-established in the United States, the move to an undergraduate degree requirement for paramedic registration has met many hurdles, largely due to the complexity of private–public funding models and interconnections with fire services.

Today, for paramedics in the United States, the National Registry of Emergency Medical Technicians (NREMT) certification is a critical component of professionalisation, providing a standardised certification process recognised across most states. However, there remains no requirement for a formal university qualification to be registered. Conversely, there is a minimum requirement of a bachelor's degree to achieve healthcare professional registration in the United Kingdom (Health and Care Profession Council), South Africa (Health Professionals Council of South Africa), Australia (Australian Health Professional Regulation Agency), and New Zealand (Te Kaunihera Manapou Paramedic Council). Furthermore, advanced specialist practice such as critical care, aeromedical rescue and retrieval, and community paramedicine often require university postgraduate qualifications up to the level of a master's degree.

The United Kingdom also saw a shift towards higher education in the late 1990s, with the establishment of paramedic degree programs at universities. The NHS played a significant role in this transition, integrating healthcare services and promoting advanced clinical training for paramedics [16].

Paramedics in Research and Academia

The role of paramedics has traditionally been associated with a mobile health response, historically focusing on the provision of primary and emergency healthcare outside the hospital environment. Over the last three decades, there has been significant evolution in the scope of paramedic practice, paralleled by emerging roles as researchers and academics. This transition reflects a broader professionalisation of paramedicine, aligning it with other health professions such as nursing and medicine, which have long embraced academic and research roles [18].

Historically, paramedic practice has relied heavily on research conducted by physicians and nurses, then used as a proxy for out-of-hospital care. Whilst this approach served its purpose, and medical and nursing researchers continue to provide vital insights for paramedic practice, it is essential that paramedic researchers contribute significantly to their own profession. Paramedicine now enjoys a robust international research profile, particularly in the United Kingdom and Australasia. Universities and ambulance services have collaborated closely with medicine, nursing, and other academic areas to produce high-quality research that informs patient care, work processes, and system efficiencies. This evolution underscores the importance of paramedics not only as practitioners but also as contributors to the body of knowledge that shapes their field [18, 19].

The transition from industry-based paramedic roles to academic positions within universities continues, driven by the need for paramedics to have the knowledge and skills necessary for a rapidly changing healthcare system. This shift is part of the ongoing professional trajectory of paramedicine. Part of the drive to embed paramedics in academia is of course through necessity. As previously noted, in South Africa, Australia, New Zealand, and the United Kingdom, paramedic education has moved into the university system, demanding academically qualified paramedics to assume teaching and research roles [20].

As the concept of paramedic-led and informed research became established through the 2000s and 2010s, the role of the paramedic as a researcher has become more clearly defined. McClelland [21] emphasises the emergence of the 'research paramedic' role, which integrates clinical practice with research responsibilities [21]. Such roles are normalised throughout the United Kingdom and are becoming more commonplace in Australia [18, 21, 22] but are yet to formally arise in the United States. To achieve parity with other healthcare progressions, the combined paramedic–researcher or clinician–academic role is essential for advancing evidence-based practices in out-of-hospital care and ensuring that paramedic services are grounded in the latest scientific evidence. The integration of research into paramedic practice helps improve patient outcomes and system efficiency, making the role of research paramedics increasingly vital [23].

The transition to academia is, however, not without challenges. Research by Munro and colleagues has revealed significant gap regarding the transition experiences of paramedics moving into academic roles. This gap highlights the need for further research to develop strategies that support paramedics in their academic careers, ensuring they are well-prepared for the demands of teaching, research, and professional development within the university setting [19, 24]. Specific challenges faced by paramedics include the need to balance clinical practice with research and teaching responsibilities, and the lack of formalised pathways for paramedics to engage in research while maintaining their clinical roles. Additionally, many paramedics recruited to academic positions lack doctoral qualifications and experience in research and publications, which can greatly contribute to academic success [18, 19].

In many cases, paramedics must choose between continuing their clinical practice and pursuing academic qualifications, often compromising their clinical careers, income, and personal time [19, 20, 23, 24]. Further, Wood [22] supports the notion that the integration of clinical research into paramedic practice is challenging, particularly in the face of a lacking workforce interest, limited buy-in by paramedics and ambulance services, and poor comprehension of evidence-based research. Wood and others identify that paramedicine is working hard to develop a research culture [22, 23]; however, this is reliant on individual paramedics engaging in research, institutional support, and better collaboration between clinicians and academic institutions. Formal research agendas have been established and are major enablers to the evolution of an advanced paramedicine research culture [25, 26].

As health system pressures build across the developed world, particularly after the coronavirus pandemic [27], workforce challenges have become pronounced. Whilst there is a documented shortage of clinicians across health, this has the potential to exacerbate the shortage of qualified paramedic academics across the United Kingdom, Australia, and New Zealand. This shortage is partly addressed by recruiting internationally, but it underscores the need for more robust domestic pathways and structured programs to develop paramedic academics [18, 23]. Such structures include formalisation of the clinician–academic model, which integrates clinical practice with academic responsibilities and is well-established in other health professions but is still developing in paramedicine. Ratifying this dual role is essential for the continued growth of the profession. It ensures that paramedics can contribute to evidence-based practice and the education of future paramedics without sacrificing their clinical expertise [18]. The clinician-academic role also brings numerous benefits, including enhanced patient care, improved healthcare systems, and increased job satisfaction for paramedics. By supporting paramedics in pursuing higher degrees and research opportunities, whilst working clinically, the profession can develop a cadre of clinician–academics who drive innovation and improvement in paramedic practice [18, 21, 22].

The evolving role of paramedics as researchers and academics is a testament to the ongoing professionalisation of the field. While significant progress has been made, particularly in the United Kingdom and Australasia, there remain challenges in supporting paramedics through this transition. Addressing these challenges requires a concerted effort to develop formalised pathways for paramedics to engage in research and academia, enable concurrent clinical practice, remove barriers to completion of higher degree by research qualifications, and assurance of essential institutional support and recognition. As the profession continues to mature, the integration of clinical practice with academic and research responsibilities will be crucial in driving paramedicine forward, ultimately enhancing patient care and advancing the profession.

Chapter Summary

Paramedicine stands on the precipice of remarkable advancement, rooted in a rich history and propelled by continuous innovation. The evolution from rudimentary first aid and transportation services to a sophisticated, evidence-based profession underscores the adaptability and appetite for growth of paramedics globally. The integration of academic rigor, advanced clinical practice, and a commitment to research has transformed paramedicine into a critical pillar of modern healthcare.

Looking forward, the profession must address the challenges of integrating clinical practice with academic responsibilities, supporting paramedics in their pursuit of higher education and research opportunities, and fostering a robust research culture. By embracing these challenges and building on the strong legacy of innovation and dedication, paramedicine will continue to advance, offering improved patient outcomes and contributing significantly to the broader healthcare landscape.

Exemplars of Paramedic-Led Research

Here are two exemplars of paramedic-led research, see Boxes 2.2 and 2.3, which showcase the progression of paramedics in research.

Box 2.2

Women's Experience of Unplanned Out-of-Hospital Birth in Paramedic Care (2019)

Research Design: A qualitative study employing narrative inquiry, collecting data through detailed interviews.

(continued)

(continued)

This study investigates the experiences of women who give birth unexpectedly before arriving at the hospital and are attended to by paramedics. Conducted in Queensland, Australia, from 2011 to 2016, the study uses a narrative inquiry methodology involving 22 narrative interviews. The research aimed to explore the perspectives of these women, highlighting the factors contributing to their out-of-hospital births and evaluating the quality of care provided by paramedics.

The study found that many women felt empowered, confident, and exhilarated during their births. However, several participants expressed concerns regarding paramedic practices, specifically citing issues such as lack of privacy, poor interpersonal skills and absence of consent for certain procedures. The narratives underscored the importance of effective communication, respect, and empathy from paramedics. Positive experiences were often linked to paramedics who displayed strong interpersonal skills and clinical competence, while negative experiences were associated with those who were perceived as disrespectful or lacking empathy.

The findings suggest several areas for improvement in paramedic care during unplanned out-of-hospital births. Recommendations include enhancing paramedic training to improve technical skills and interpersonal communication, ensuring privacy, and emphasising the importance of obtaining informed consent. The study highlights the need for a patient-centred approach that respects women's autonomy and involves them in decision-making processes.

Source: Adapted from [28]

Box 2.3

Effect of a Resuscitation Quality Improvement Programme on Outcomes from Out-of-hospital Cardiac Arrest (2021)

Research Design: Interrupted time-series analysis

This study evaluated the impact of a resuscitation quality improvement programme on survival outcomes following out-of-hospital cardiac arrest (OHCA). Researchers compared two periods: a control period (January 2015–January 2019) before the programme's implementation and an intervention period (February 2019–January 2020) after the high-performance CPR programme was introduced. The study aimed to assess improvements in survival to hospital discharge, event survival, and return of spontaneous circulation (ROSC).

A total of 10,600 OHCA patients of medical origin were included, with 8,270 in the control period and 2,330 in the intervention period. Following the implementation of high-performance CPR, adjusted odds ratios (AOR) showed statistically significant increases in survival outcomes. Monthly survival to hospital discharge increased by 50% (AOR 1.50; 95% CI: 1.10, 2.04; p = 0.01), while event survival improved by 34% (AOR 1.34; 95% CI: 1.09, 1.65; p = 0.006), and ROSC rose by 38% (AOR 1.38; 95% CI: 1.14, 1.65; p = 0.001). When removing the non-significant temporal trend, the overall risk-adjusted odds of survival over the 12-month intervention period showed a 33% increase (AOR 1.33; 95% CI: 1.11, 1.58; p = 0.002).

Source: Adapted from [29].

Conclusion

With a legacy of frontline care and emerging academic contribution, paramedicine is positioned to drive further advancements in clinical and research domains. As the profession integrates more deeply into the academic and healthcare landscape, challenges remain. These include balancing clinical and academic roles, fostering a robust research culture, and supporting paramedics in higher education pursuits. These hurdles, while significant, represent opportunities to strengthen the profession.

Paramedicine's journey forward will be marked by embracing these challenges and fostering a culture of continuous learning and adaptation. By supporting clinician–academics, advancing evidence-based practice, and promoting interdisciplinary collaboration, the field will continue to enhance patient outcomes and solidify its place as an essential, dynamic pillar within the healthcare system.

References

1. Cole, P.J. (1996). The Military Orders in War and Peace. *The International History Review* 18 (3): 620–628.

2. Pollock, A. (2015). Historical perspectives in the ambulance service. In: *Ambulance Services: Leadership and Management Perspectives* (ed. P. Wankhade and K. Mackway-Jones), 17–28. Springer.

3. Pozner, C.N., Zane, R., Nelson, S.J., and Levine, M. (2004). International EMS systems: The United States: past, present, and future. *Resuscitation* 60 (3): 239–244.

4. Makrides, T., Ross, L., Gosling, C. et al. (2022). From stretcher bearer to practitioner: a brief narrative review of the history of

the Anglo-American paramedic system. *Australasian Emergency Care* 25 (4): 347–353.

5. Allison, C.E. and Trunkey, D.D. (2009). Battlefield trauma, traumatic shock and consequences: war-related advances in critical care. *Critical Care Clinics* 25 (1): 31–45.

6. Penn-Barwell, J.G., Roberts, S.A., Midwinter, M.J., and Bishop, J.R. (2015). Improved survival in UK combat casualties from Iraq and Afghanistan: 2003–2012. *Journal of Trauma and Acute Care Surgery* 78 (5): 1014–1020.

7. Pantridge, J.F. and Wilson, C. (1996). A history of prehospital coronary care. *The Ulster Medical Journal* 65 (1): 68.

8. Edwards, M.L. (2019). Pittsburgh's Freedom House Ambulance Service: the origins of emergency medical services and the politics of race and health. *Journal of the History of Medicine and Allied Sciences* 74 (4): 440–466.

9. Caroline, N.L. and Elling, B. (2013). *Nancy Caroline's Emergency Care in the Streets*. Jones & Bartlett Publishers.

10. World Bank (2021). *The State of Emergency Medical Services in Sub-Saharan Africa*. World Bank.

11. Reed, B., Cowin, L., O'Meara, P., and Wilson, I. (2022). A qualitative exploration of the perceptions of professional registration by Australian paramedics during the transition into professional regulation. *Medical Law International* 22 (4): 327–348.

12. Dickison, P., Hostler, D., Platt, T.E., and Wang, H.E. (2006). Program accreditation effect on paramedic credentialing examination success rate. *Prehospital Emergency Care* 10 (2): 224–228.

13. Williams, B., Onsman, A., and Brown, T. (2009). From stretcher-bearer to paramedic: the Australian paramedics' move towards professionalisation. *Australasian Journal of Paramedicine* 7: 1–12.

14. Brooks, I.A., Grantham, H., Spencer, C., and Archer, F. (2018). A review of the literature: the transition of entry-level paramedic education in Australia from vocational to higher education (1961–2017). *Australasian Journal of Paramedicine* 15: 1–11.

15. Brooks, I.A., Sayre, M.R., Spencer, C., and Archer, F.L. (2016). An historical examination of the development of emergency medical services education in the US through key reports (1966–2014). *Prehospital and Disaster Medicine* 31 (1): 90–97.

16. Brooks, I.A., Cooke, M., Spencer, C., and Archer, F. (2016). A review of key national reports to describe the development of paramedic education in England (1966–2014). *Emergency Medicine Journal* 33 (12): 876–881.

17. O'Brien, K., Moore, A., Dawson, D., and Hartley, P. (2014). An Australian story: paramedic education and practice in transition. *Australasian Journal of Paramedicine* 11: 1–13.

18. Meadley, B.N., Andrews, T., Delardes, B.J., and Shannon, B.P. (2022). The evolution of clinician-academics in paramedicine: completing the picture of professionalism. *Prehospital and Disaster Medicine* 37 (5): 574–576.

19. Munro, G., O'Meara, P., and Kenny, A. (2016). Paramedic transition into an academic role in universities: a scoping review. *Journal of Paramedic Practice* 8 (9): 452–457.

20. Munro GG, O'Meara P, Mathisen B. Paramedic transition into an academic role in universities: A qualitative survey of paramedic academics in Australia and New Zealand. *Irish Journal of Paramedicine* 2019; 4(1). doi: https://doi.org/10.32378/ijp.v4i1.107.

21. McClelland, G. (2013). The research paramedic: a new role. *Journal of Paramedic Practice* 5 (10): 582–586.

22. Wood, K. (2012). Integrating clinical research into paramedic practice: current trends and influences. *Journal of Paramedic Practice* 4 (9): 502–508.

23. Runacres, J., Harvey, H., O'Brien, S., and Halck, A. (2024). Paramedics as researchers: a systematic review of paramedic perspectives of engaging in research activity from training to practice. *The Journal of Emergency Medicine* 66 (6): e680–e689.

24. Munro, G.G., O'Meara, P., and Mathisen, B. (2018). Paramedic academics in Australia and New Zealand: the 'no man's land' of professional identity. *Nurse Education in Practice* 33: 33–36.

25. O'Meara, P., Maguire, B., Jennings, P., and Simpson, P. (2015). Building an Australasian paramedicine research agenda: a narrative review. *Health Research and Policy System* 13: 79.

26. Pap, R., Barr, N., Hutchison, A. et al. (2024). Research agenda and priorities for Australian and New Zealand paramedicine: a Delphi consensus study. *Paramedicine* 21 (3): 94–107.

27. Agyeman-Manu, K., Ghebreyesus, T.A., Maait, M. et al. (2023). Prioritising the health and care workforce shortage: protect, invest, together. *The Lancet Global Health* 11 (8): e1162–e1164.

28. Flanagan, B., Lord, B., Reed, R., and Crimmins, G. (2019). Women's experience of unplanned out-of-hospital birth in paramedic care. *BMC Emergency Medicine* 19: 1–7.

29. Nehme, Z., Ball, J., Stephenson, M. et al. (2021). Effect of a resuscitation quality improvement programme on outcomes from out-of-hospital cardiac arrest. *Resuscitation* 162: 236–244.

Further Reading

Makrides, T., Ross, L., Gosling, C. et al. (2022). From stretcher bearer to practitioner: a brief narrative review of the history of the Anglo-American paramedic system. *Australasian Emergency Care* 25 (4): 347–353.

Meadley, B.N., Andrews, T., Delardes, B.J., and Shannon, B.P. (2022). The evolution of clinician-academics in paramedicine: completing the picture of professionalism. *Prehospital and Disaster Medicine* 37 (5): 574–576.

Newton, A., Hunt, B., and Williams, J. (2020). The paramedic profession: disruptive innovation and barriers to further progress. *Journal of Paramedic Practice* 12 (4): 138–148.

Shannon, B., Baldry, S., O'Meara, P. et al. (2023). The definition of a community paramedic: an international consensus. *Paramedicine* 20 (1): 4–22.

Chapter 3
Education

Brendan Shannon and Alan Michael Batt

Department of Paramedicine, Monash University, Melbourne, Victoria, Australia

Chapter Objectives

1. Outline the progression of paramedicine education from undergraduate to doctoral levels.
2. Evaluate the role of the clinician–academic pathway and its impact on the integration of clinical practice and research.

Research-focused Careers for Paramedics, First Edition.
Edited by Gregory A. Whitley and Scott Munro.
© 2025 John Wiley & Sons Ltd. Published 2025 by John Wiley & Sons Ltd.

3. Describe the various types of paramedicine education programs and the specific requirements and expectations at each level of study.
4. Discuss the challenges and benefits of pursuing full-time versus part-time study.
5. Identify key considerations in selecting a research topic and developing a doctoral proposal.
6. Explain the importance of mentorship, networking, and supervision in developing a successful research career in paramedicine.

Introduction

An analogy offered by Petre and Rugge [1] likens undertaking a PhD to a cabinetmaking apprenticeship. Over the course of the apprenticeship, the apprentice learns and demonstrates that they have acquired certain knowledge and skills related to cabinetmaking. Others offered that this analogy can be applied to all levels of research within paramedicine, not just the PhD [2]. Applying the analogy to an undergraduate bachelor's degree, the student learns the fundamentals of cabinetmaking—such as where to find materials (*can access research findings*), what materials are appropriate (*uses reliable sources*), and the foundations of assembling a cabinet (*understands the elements of reliable research*). Moving to a master's degree, the learner develops an intermediate understanding of making a cabinet—such as demonstrating how to assemble various components in a cabinet under supervision (*understands and implements various research designs*), how to critique an assembled cabinet (*performs critical appraisal*), and how to improve the next cabinet (*links findings to practice and future directions).* Finally, in a doctoral context, the doctoral student demonstrates the knowledge and skills required to be a cabinetmaker *(has the skills required to be an independent researcher),* whereby they demonstrate their ability to source materials, plan, and build a new cabinet *(conducts research that produces new knowledge)* that ultimately passes the scrutiny of their master craftsman *(conducts trustworthy research that passes examination and meets the conventions of the field).*

To fully embrace this analogy, the importance of education and mentoring in developing research careers for paramedics becomes clear. Those who wish to pursue a career in research must progress from foundational knowledge of the research process to expertise in conducting research and translating findings, via a form of 'apprenticeship'. However, it can be a challenge to make sense of all the choices and pathways that now exist. You might have found yourself asking *"What program should I choose?", "Do I need a PhD to do research?",* and *"Is it possible to study while working?".* These and many other questions are often posed by those interested in pursuing a research career in paramedicine. Unfortunately, the answers are often elusive, and where answers are found, they can be incomplete, inaccessible, or isolated from career progression choices. Until this chapter that is. Therefore, this chapter seeks to (i) provide advice on the foundational elements of pursuing a research career in paramedicine, (ii) outline various education programme choices, (iii) offer insights into the requirements and expectations at each level of study, (iv) provide structure to determining research topics, and (v) demonstrate the relationship between education and other elements of your professional life in developing your research career.

Early Considerations

Undergraduate Research/Evidence-Based Practice Module

First things first: you do not need to be a research professional or hold a PhD to access and appreciate research findings. Including foundational research teachings in undergraduate education is essential to develop a generation of paramedics who can find, understand, and use research findings in their practice. Learners have questions—many questions! These questions should be encouraged, and you must learn a logical, structured process by which to best answer them. Student-led research contributes to improved evidence-based practice [3], and undergraduate research participants are more likely to pursue graduate education and additional research activity in their future careers [4]. Evidence from student-led research programs in Australia, the United Kingdom, and Canada supports the ability of undergraduate learners to contribute meaningfully to the paramedic profession's body of knowledge [5–8]. For example, some of the first research into paramedic students' attitudes towards people experiencing homelessness came from undergraduate paramedic students in Canada and Australia [9, 10].

Publishing as a Student (CPD Articles, Literature Reviews)

One of the first forays into research for many learners is the need to perform a literature review, or a review of the evidence within their clinical courses. However, a word of caution. Requiring learners to perform this activity without adequate support can result in negative perceptions of research activity. This can be due to feeling over-burdened, feeling lost in the process due to lacking core knowledge and skills, and thus being unable to produce meaningful results. Keeping activities small in scope, providing adequate resources and support, and encouraging collaborative efforts can go some way towards creating a positive experience. In addition, this will likely improve the quality of the output, which may then be considered for dissemination. Publishing student-led work can present challenges due to sample sizes, logistical constraints, and a lack of appropriate venues. However, these challenges can be overcome by collaborating with academics who can provide mentoring and guidance. Additionally, consider contributing to student-led conferences, poster presentations, trade magazines, and other outlets, not just peer-reviewed journals.

Networking

Networking is likely the least talked about and yet one of the most important elements of any successful research career. Get out there—go to conferences, attend online events, volunteer to help with studies, and talk to people. A level of 'professional boldness' is required when approaching networking [11]. It matters not whether you are an undergraduate student or a senior academic—encourage all within the profession to contact others, across boundaries and borders, nationally and internationally. While workloads and other commitments may mean that not all connections result in an immediate ability to collaborate, the first step to any fruitful collaboration and relationship is simply making the connection.

The Clinician–Academic Pathway

The clinician–academic pathway in paramedicine is emerging internationally, with the United Kingdom leading with hybrid roles combining clinical and academic elements [12]. Similar roles exist in Australia and Canada but are still in their infancy. Despite advancements in paramedic-led research, formalised pathways supporting concurrent research and clinical practice are rare. Unlike other health professions with established clinician–academic positions, paramedics face limited flexibility in part-time clinical roles due to operational demands. [13] Those pursuing higher degrees by research (HDR) often compromise their clinical careers, income, or personal time. The clinician–academic role is crucial for implementing research outcomes, requiring both clinical practice and research understanding. Formalizing this role involves recognizing it with titles and providing support through workplace schemes for balanced research and clinical duties, along with appropriate remuneration. This alignment with other health professions will offer additional career paths, enhance healthcare systems [14], and improve job satisfaction, benefiting paramedics, the profession, and patients. As this role solidifies within career pathways, it will become highly sought after, but it begins with a strong educational foundation.

Bachelor's-Level Study

Bachelor's-level study in paramedicine is an advanced technical knowledge in paramedic practice, involving a critical understanding of the key principles. Paramedic education across multiple countries has recently shifted towards bachelor's degree requirements for entry-to-practice. Across national qualifications frameworks this equates to level 6 (United Kingdom), levels 7–8 (Ireland, Australia, New Zealand), and levels 9–10 (Scotland).

Pre-registration Bachelors

Pre-registration bachelor's degrees are not the focus of this chapter, but it would be remiss to not mention them. These degrees are largely targeted at creating a competent paramedic clinician for entry into the clinical workforce. Recent shifts towards creating a more holistic paramedic are to be welcomed, and indeed, it is often the first exposure to areas of paramedicine such as research and education in these education programmes that lays a foundation for future engagement.

Bachelors Top-up Degrees

Existing vocationally qualified paramedics (e.g., higher diploma, diploma, and certificate holders) who wish to further their education can often access 'top-up' degrees. These are commonly 18–24 months in duration and focus on non-technical, professional, and/or advanced clinical learning. These types of degrees can often be completed via fully online or hybrid models. If you are an existing vocationally qualified paramedic, these programmes provide a means by which to advance your education and position yourself for entry to higher degrees.

Honours Bachelor's Degrees

Honours bachelor's degrees come in two main formats. The first is a direct programme that results in a paramedic qualification, along with the completion of a capstone project or dissertation/thesis. The second is a one-year programme that is available to those with a bachelor's degree (or equivalent), that is an intensive research-focused degree with a thesis element.

The Gap Between Bachelor- and Master's-Level Study

A key difference between undergraduate- and graduate-level study is the ability to synthesise information from multiple sources and reflect on its application to support decision-making. For example, a master's qualified paramedic can take information from published literature, clinical guidelines, education, and reflections on previous experience and combine them to inform case management decisions.

Master's-Level Study

Master's-level study in paramedicine is the critical awareness of issues and highly specialised knowledge of the field and practice of paramedicine. Across national qualifications frameworks, this equates to level 7 (United Kingdom), level 9 (Ireland, Australia, New Zealand), and level 11 (Scotland).

Types of Master's Degree

Where to start here? There are so many choices when it comes to master's degrees. Using the combined categories from several paramedic career frameworks, there are five broad categories of master's degrees that you might find relevant—master's degrees in clinical practice, leadership and management, education, research, and policy. Within these categories, you will find a multitude of distinct offerings, and the exact title or degree award can vary significantly (see **Table 3.1**). For example, if you were interested in pursuing a master's degree in education, you will find there are Master of Education (MEd), Master of Science in Health Professions Education (MSc HPE), and Master of Arts in Education (MAEd) degrees to choose from to name but a few. The same is true for research—research-focused master's degrees have a multitude of different titles and academic awards.

In general, the distinction between titles and awards will come down to one main characteristic—whether it is a taught programme or a research programme. You will need to consider this if you intend to pursue future doctoral studies, as many taught programmes do not meet the entry requirements for doctoral admissions. Coursework-only master's degrees without a research component will often not be acceptable for entry to doctoral programmes.

Selecting a Topic of Research

Selecting a research topic is a crucial step in the research process, often initiated by a curious mind. For paramedics and paramedic students, research questions typically arise from practical experiences and a desire to improve clinical practices. These questions can stem from clinical conundrums encountered in the field, prompting reflection on whether current methods are optimal. Observing different interventions or processes in various settings may inspire further

Table 3.1 Variation in qualification across the pillars of professional practice

	Clinical practice	Leadership and management	Education	Research	Policy
Sample degree awards—master's level	Master of Science in Advanced Clinical Practice (MSc) Master of Paramedicine	Master of Arts in Leadership (MA) Master of Health Management (MHM) Master of Health Administration (MHA) Master of Business Administration (MBA)	Master of Education (MEd) MSc in Health Professions Education (MSc) MSc in Medical Education Master of Educational Technology (MET)	MSc in Research Master of Clinical Research (MClinRes) Master of Research (MRes) Master of Letters (MLitt) Master of Philosophy (MPhil)	Master of Public Policy (MPP) Master of Public Health (MPH) Master of Laws (LLM)
Sample degree awards—doctoral level	Professional doctorate (DProf) Doctor of Advanced Clinical Practice Doctor of Philosophy (PhD/DPhil)	Professional doctorate (DProf) Doctor of Business Administration (DBA) Doctor of Philosophy (PhD/DPhil)	Professional doctorate (DProf) Doctor of Education (EdD) Doctor of Philosophy (PhD/DPhil)	Doctor of Philosophy (PhD/DPhil)	Professional doctorate (DProf) Doctor of Philosophy (PhD/DPhil)

investigation to enhance one's own practice area. Additionally, paramedics are often driven by the need for purpose and efficiency in their work, leading them to question and seek improvements in systems, processes, or interventions. Lastly, opportunities for grants or external inspiration from academic supervisors or stakeholders such as health services can also spark research interest.

Once a potential research idea is identified, it's essential to take a step back and follow a structured approach to ensure success and worthy of your time. The initial step involves seeking feedback from experts in the field to assess the feasibility and relevance of the research idea. Engaging with accessible experts, including university based researchers and professionals within paramedicine or wider, helps to refine the idea and provides valuable feedback. It is crucial to determine whether the research has been previously investigated and gauge the interest of key stakeholders to support your topic, sometimes despite all your passion you must be willing to let go and move to something else to ensure you can undertake the research. A brief scan of existing literature, both published and grey, helps to contextualise the research idea within the current body of knowledge [15]—there is no point researching something that's already been answered or may be inundated with researchers. This preliminary exploration aids in understanding the key concepts and identifying gaps that the research could address. Involving stakeholders early, including research mentors and relevant organisations, ensures that the research has the necessary support and aligns with practical needs while still being achievable within the time constraints of a master's-level research program.

The Gap Between Master's- and Doctoral-Level Study

The key differences between master's- and doctoral-level study are an ability to use theoretical and conceptual foundations to frame questions, the ability to generate new knowledge, and the ability to link disparate pieces of evidence to gain new insights. For example, a doctoral-educated paramedic can make connections between theoretical approaches used in other disciplines (e.g., social work, engineering) and their novel application to solve issues in paramedicine (e.g., how to think about practice). While a master's degree can be akin to assembling a piece of prefabricated furniture, where the student's role involves putting together the pieces of the puzzle, doctoral-level study is more like being given a collection of raw materials and being tasked with carving and creating the furniture from scratch—while being guided and supported by experienced mentors of course!

Doctoral-Level Study

Doctoral-level study in paramedicine is the creation and use of knowledge at the most advanced frontier of the paramedicine profession. Across national qualifications frameworks, this equates to level 8 (United Kingdom), level 10 (Ireland, Australia, New Zealand), and level 12 (Scotland).

Should I Do a PhD/DPhil or a Professional Doctorate?

It simply comes down to what you hope to achieve with and after the qualification. PhDs are more commonly undertaken by those who want to pursue a research-intense career pathway, often within or conjoint with an academic appointment. Meanwhile, professional doctorates are often completed by those who wish to focus on a specific area of practice, with an improvement lens. Professional practice is at the heart of a professional doctorate programme, as the aim of these programmes is to develop researching professionals rather than professional researchers [16].

Developing a Doctoral Research Application/Proposal

Developing a doctoral research application or proposal involves several steps that span logistical, conceptual, and administrative aspects. Each step is essential to ensure a comprehensive and well-prepared application that meets the standards of doctoral programs and proves to a potential supervisory team that your research is necessary, meaningful, and worthy of their investment. Logistically, the first step is to research various universities and programs to find one that aligns with your research interests and career goals. Consider the reputation of the program, faculty expertise, available resources, and the university's support for doctoral candidates. Identifying potential supervisors whose research interests align with yours is crucial, as a good supervisor provides essential guidance, support, and mentorship throughout your doctoral journey. Additionally, exploring funding options, including scholarships and grants, is necessary particularly if you are looking to secure financial support to cover tuition fees, research costs, and living expenses as these will vary across different countries. Assessing how to balance doctoral studies with personal and professional responsibilities through effective time management and a strong support system is also important.

Conceptually, choosing a research topic that addresses a significant gap in existing knowledge and has the potential to contribute meaningfully to the field of paramedicine is vital. Clearly articulating why pursuing a PhD is the right path for your research and career goals, and explaining how it fits into your long-term plans, helps establish a strong rationale. Developing a detailed research plan that outlines your research question, objectives, methodology, and expected outcomes demonstrates the feasibility of your research and your ability to carry it out successfully. By showcasing how your research will make a meaningful contribution to the field, you can prove to the supervisory team that their investment in your research will be worthwhile.

Administratively, ensuring that you meet all prerequisites for the doctoral program, including academic qualifications, relevant experience, and language proficiency if applicable, is important. You don't want an administrative oversight to be the pillar that falls resulting in a waste of time and effort by all involved. By addressing these steps and demonstrating a well-thought-out and feasible research plan, you can develop a robust doctoral research application that proves to your potential supervisory team that your research is necessary, meaningful, and worthy of their investment.

Selecting a Topic

Ideally, you will study something that is valuable and of interest to you, the profession, and can make a meaningful impact (e.g., on patient outcomes, on paramedic wellbeing). Depending on how you approach this, this might be a topic within an existing project or program of research (e.g., a funded PhD opportunity in stroke care), a topic that you have previously researched and wish to pursue further, or a topic that you have never studied before. Whichever route you take, the following insights may prove helpful:

- Try to get to the root cause or higher-order issue. What you initially determine to be a clinical practice issue may, for example, be influenced by curriculum design, health policy, or national frameworks. Sometimes the thing you think you're interested in is just an example of a deeper issue that may pique your interest. For example, you might be interested in addressing emergency department handover delays and assume that the primary cause is the increasing demand from patients with lower acuity needs. However, when you dig deeper, you might discover that these patients do not significantly contribute to the delays. Instead, the root cause might lie in hospital discharge delays, lack of bed availability, or a broader breakdown in the primary care system. These issues are often influenced by larger systemic factors, including funding policies, health system structures, and a societal trend towards immediate care for all health needs. Getting to this higher-order thinking is best achieved by abstracting and approaching your topic from different theoretical perspectives [17]. Try on some different paradigms and perspectives to see which fits best for you.
- Read broadly (outside of paramedicine, across disciplines), then read deeply (go down rabbit holes to see which interests you most), then read some more (all the while looking for connections, gaps, and opportunities in the literature).

- Write as you go. There's an old Irish saying that says *"you can't plough a field by turning it over in your mind."* Similarly, you can't write a PhD thesis without writing. Do it as you go, and it will help to clarify your thinking.
- Be open to changing and evolving your topic. It's ok not to know exactly what you are doing in a PhD. It's also ok to be led by your findings and change your plan incrementally and iteratively.

Selecting a Supervisory Team

Selecting the right supervisory team is a crucial step in ensuring the success of your doctoral research. The right team not only guides you through the complexities of your research but also supports your academic and professional development. However, there are specific challenges in the academic workforce within paramedicine that need careful consideration. One of the primary challenges is the limited availability of subject matter experts within the paramedicine field available to supervise doctoral students [18]. It may be necessary to seek outside supervision from experts in related disciplines to ensure you have the necessary guidance and knowledge. While it might be tempting to pursue supervision from well-known or 'big name' academics, it's important to consider their availability and commitment. Often, these individuals may lack the time to provide the dedicated support and mentorship required for your doctoral journey. Your supervisory team should be supportive, available, and committed to your success. They should provide critical insights into contemporary issues in the field, highlight opportunities within existing research, and potentially give you access to valuable resources such as data and funding. This support can significantly narrow your research focus and enhance the quality and impact of your work.

Finding the right supervisory team involves careful consideration of several factors. Firstly, look for supervisors whose research interests align with your own. This alignment ensures that they have the expertise and enthusiasm to support your work. Secondly, assess their track record in supervising doctoral candidates, successful supervisors typically have a history of guiding students to completion. Thirdly, consider their accessibility and willingness to meet regularly, as consistent communication is key to progressing your research. Moreover, a good supervisory team brings diverse perspectives and expertise to your project. Consider forming a team with members from different backgrounds who can offer varied insights and approaches to your research question [19]. This diversity can enrich your research and help you navigate interdisciplinary challenges. It's also important to note that you should be open to bringing new supervisors and researchers into the team for certain aspects of your research as needed, particularly if they bring experience or expertise in certain methodologies the existing team does not have.

Full-Time Versus Part-Time Study

Pre-registration degrees are commonly completed full time, while top-up degrees are for the most part completed part time. This affords opportunities for existing paramedics to continue to work, while furthering their education. However, some scholarships and financial support schemes are only available to full-time students, or those employed less than a certain number of hours per week, so make sure you consider this when deciding on your mode of study. In addition, hybrid programmes may require your attendance on campus, so factor in additional travel costs as well as other considerations (e.g., time off work, childcare).

Choosing between full-time and part-time master's and doctoral degrees is a significant decision that can impact your academic experience, professional life, and personal commitments. Each option has its advantages and challenges, and the best choice depends on individual circumstances, goals, and resources. Opting for full time often allows for a more immersive and focused academic experience. As a full-time student, you can dedicate most of your time to your studies, potentially completing the program faster. This option is beneficial for those who aim to swiftly transition to advanced roles, academic roles, or pursue further studies, without prolonged interruptions. Full-time study can be easier to balance as you can treat it as your job and protect your time outside of your study.

However, full-time study also comes with challenges like financial strain, as students may face difficulties without the ability to work full time, requiring strong time management skills to balance intensive coursework with personal life [20]. Moreover, full-time study may necessitate taking a break from professional clinical roles, potentially impacting career progression and income. Full time also requires sacrifices, that may be different, such as loss of professional identity, seniority, pension, loss of pay, and risk of non-completion. It's important to note the student contract you may sign at your chosen institution can sometimes limit the amount of paid work outside of the study you commit to undertake, typically 15–20 hours/week is a suggested limit.

A part-time degree offers flexibility, allowing paramedics to continue working while studying. This option is particularly appealing to paramedics who wish to advance their education without pausing their careers. This option balances work, study, and personal life, providing practical experience and financial stability. However, it may delay career advancement and limit campus engagement and networking opportunities. While part-time study is achievable, it still requires sacrifices related to time management, impact on hobbies and free time activities, and balancing home and life commitments.

During the education journey, students in both full-time and part-time pathways may find themselves envious of the advantages enjoyed by the other. Part-time students might envy the rapid completion times and the singular focus that full-time students can dedicate to their research. Conversely, full-time students might be envious of the extended timelines that part-time students have, which can alleviate the pressure of delays beyond their control, such as lengthy publication peer review processes, ethics review timelines, accessibility to data, and prolonged recruitment periods.

Dealing with Difficult Times

Regardless of whether you choose full-time or part-time study, life continues, and you will be faced with both good times and difficult times. Uncertainty around your research question, challenges with recruitment, demanding peer review reports, and failing to secure funding grants may place stress on you within your studies. In addition to the demands of your education, personal health, family issues, parenting responsibilities, and financial situations can all impact your well-being and productivity. It is crucial to prioritise rest and self-care. Don't feel guilty about taking vacations or breaks to handle personal matters. Life inevitably happens during any degree, and it's important to manage these occurrences effectively.

It's also important to be aware that the stress of pursuing higher education can sometimes lead to more serious mental health challenges, such as anxiety and depression. This is especially true in environments where there are strained relationships with supervisors, unclear processes, overwhelming workloads, uncertainty about future career prospects and financial pressures [21]. Recognising these potential stressors and seeking support early can make a significant difference in maintaining your well-being throughout your studies. With that in mind, clearly communicate with your supervisors and be sure to access all university supports that are available to you. Having a support group of other paramedics pursuing education can be an enormous benefit, and with current technology, these groups can be convened virtually across borders and oceans. Finally, be kind to yourself. Everyone faces difficult times when undertaking long journeys. Keep track of each little victory, as these eventually become larger victories, culminating in you eventually crossing the finish line. Remember that everyone's journey looks different, so don't fall victim to comparing your progress to others.

Different Routes to the Same Destination

Brendan: In my early 20s, as paramedicine evolved towards degree-entry pathways in most ambulance services in Australia, I pursued a traditional pre-registration bachelor's degree in paramedicine. After completing my degree, I immediately entered clinical practice. During this time, I spent considerable time dealing with ED access delays [22], sparking my curiosity about the causes and solutions. Instead of pursuing a clinical-based master's degree for an advanced practice role in critical care as I had initially planned, I chose to undertake a standalone honours degree part-time while working full-time to explore research and address the ED access issue. Fortunately, good mentorship during my honour's degree enabled me to achieve a high mark and enrol in a PhD program. I pursued my PhD part-time due to family responsibilities and a mortgage, requiring full-time employment. Over six years, I balanced a growing clinical and academic career while making significant sacrifices to home life, supported by my family. My path, guided by curiosity and not exactly meticulously planned out, led me to become a tenured academic at a highly ranked institution. My tertiary academic journey has spanned 12 years of study over 16 years.

Alan: I am a vocationally trained paramedic, and I hold a diploma—I never completed a bachelor's degree. I immediately entered clinical practice after completing my diploma, and four years later began the journey to becoming an educator. During my time as a paramedic educator across several countries, I noticed a disconnect between the realities of practice, and how we prepared learners. Several postgraduate degrees later (in clinical practice and medical education), this eventually led me to undertake a PhD to explore and improve the link between the realities of practice and education programmes. I completed my PhD in four years (two years part-time and two years full-time) while balancing home life and work commitments. All told, my academic journey took over 15 years to complete. I am now an academic at highly ranked institutions in Australia and Canada and supervise several postgraduate students in (and outside of) paramedicine. Like Brendan, my path was carved largely by curiosity and was in only the very loosest terms 'planned'.

After the Degree

Paramedicine would benefit greatly from a healthy pool of paramedics who want to contribute to the future of the profession through continuing academic activities [23]. Such a future faces challenges due to a lack of appropriately designated and funded positions, the disconnect often evident between academic institutions and ambulance services, and a lack of investment in strengthening the research and development lens of the profession in general. Research broadly is underfunded and highly competitive, a reality faced by many health professions globally. Yet as paramedicine develops its distinct research body, master's and PhD holders are in high demand to supervise the next generation of researchers. This situation presents a unique challenge: the limited pool of paramedicine researchers often finds themselves quickly thrust into research or educational leadership positions, leaving little room for their own growth. Being selective in research projects and supervision is crucial for building expertise and becoming a content specialist. This selectivity also provides opportunities to contribute to developing new researchers, who will, in turn, give back to the research community.

Supervising the Next Generation

Supervising and mentoring students enables experienced researchers to learn and grow while giving back to the community. Teaching and mentoring solidifies one's knowledge and guides students through the research process, helping them build their skills. This mentorship reminds researchers of their progress, and a compassionate and encouraging approach to supervision goes a long way. Teaching students to write, analyse, and conduct research with proper foundations, while being supported by other researchers, will continue to grow the profession's research capacity. By supporting and mentoring the next generation of researchers, we can ensure the continued advancement and development of paramedicine. This approach will create a sustainable cycle of knowledge and expertise, ultimately benefiting the entire profession and improving the communities we serve.

Some Final Thoughts

The journey of undertaking education potentially culminating in the completion of a PhD can seem daunting and, at times, impossible. However, remember that many have walked this path before you, and if they can do it, so can you. It won't always be smooth sailing, but it will lead to experiences and opportunities you never imagined, and you may find yourself leaving the world a better place. Embracing the challenge of further education can open doors to paths in life and experiences you never anticipated, offering the potential to make significant contributions to the field and beyond. So, take that first step and let your curiosity guide you.

> "You don't have to see the whole staircase, just take the first step."
>
> —Martin Luther King Jr.
> (paraphrased by Marian Wright Edelman)

Conclusion

This chapter has explored the journey from undergraduate education to doctoral-level research in paramedicine. We have highlighted the importance of education, mentoring, and choosing the right supervisory team, as well as the practical considerations of balancing full-time and part-time study throughout. The journey through education can be challenging but is deeply rewarding, offering the opportunity to make significant contributions to the field and improve communities. Remember, every step you take brings you closer to your goals, and your dedication to research and education will help advance not just yourself but the paramedicine profession overall.

References

1. Petre, M. and Rugg, G. (2010). *The Unwritten Rules Of PhD Research*. McGraw-Hill Education (UK) 288p.
2. Batt, A.M. and Knox, S. (2017). Building research capacity among Irish prehospital practitioners. *Irish Journal of Paramedicine* 2 (2): 2–5.

3. Strong, G. and Thompson, S. (2016). Student enquiry: the power of student research to influence evidence-based. *Whitireia Nursing and Health Journal* 23: 21–23.

4. Hathaway, R.S., Nagda, B.A., and Gregerman, S.R. (2002). The relationship of undergraduate research participation to graduate and professional education pursuit: an empirical study. *Journal of College Student Development* 43 (5): 614–631.

5. Batt, A.M., Steary, D., Mason, P. et al. (2019). The students are our future: growing the next generation of paramedic researchers in Canada. *Canadian Paramedicine* 42 (4): 12–15.

6. Boyle, M. (2015). Promoting the next wave of paramedic researchers. *Australasian Journal of Paramedicine* 12 (4): 4–5.

7. O'Meara, P. (2014). Student research: the future of paramedicine. *Australasian Journal of Paramedicine* 11 (5): 11–13.

8. Smith G. The importance of student paramedic contributions to prehospital research. *Australasian Journal of Paramedicine* 2015; 12(4). doi: https://doi.org/10.33151/ajp.12.4.488.

9. Cochrane, A., Pithia, P., Laird, E. et al. (2019). Investigating the attitudes of Canadian paramedic students towards homelessness. *International Journal of Caring Sciences* 12 (3): 1781–1787.

10. Prakash, S., Brown, S., Murphy, M., and Williams, B. (2020). Paramedic student empathetic attitudes towards homelessness: a mixed methods pilot study. *International Journal of Emergency Services* 9 (3): 273–282.

11. Simpson, P. (2024). Leveraging collaboration to enhance quality in paramedicine research. *Paramedicine* 21 (4): 144–146.

12. McClelland, G. (2013). The research paramedic: a new role. *Journal of Paramedic Practice* 5 (10): 582–586.

13. Meadley, B.N., Andrews, T., Delardes, B.J., and Shannon, B.P. (2022). The evolution of clinician-academics in paramedicine: completing the picture of professionalism. *Prehospital and Disaster Medicine* 37 (5): 574–576.

14. Olswang, L.B. and Prelock, P.A. (2015). Bridging the gap between research and practice: implementation science. *Journal of Speech, Language, and Hearing Research* 58 (6): S1818–S1826.

15. Charlton, P., Doucet, S., Azar, R. et al. (2019). The use of the environmental scan in health services delivery research: a scoping review protocol. *BMJ Open* 9 (9): e029805.

16. Halliwell, D. (2001). Professional doctorates for paramedics: a personal journey. *Journal of Paramedic Practice* 2 (2).

17. Brydges, M. and Batt, A.M. (2023). Untangling the web: the need for theory, theoretical frameworks, and conceptual frameworks in paramedic research. *Paramedicine* 20 (4): 89–93.

18. Ross, L., Reynolds, L., Reeves, H. et al. (2023 Jul). Barriers and enablers to paramedicine research in Australasia—A cross-sectional survey. *Paramedicine* 20 (4): 107–116.

19. Borregaard, B., Massouh, A., Hendriks, J. et al. (2022). The X-factors of PhD supervision: ACNAP top 10 tips on choosing a PhD supervisor. *European Journal of Cardiovascular Nursing* 21 (5): 399–401.

20. Cohen, M.A.O. and Greenberg, S. (2011). The struggle to succeed: factors associated with the persistence of part-time adult students seeking a Master's degree. *Continuing Higher Education Review* 75: 101–112.

21. Mackie, S.A. and Bates, G.W. (2019). Contribution of the doctoral education environment to PhD candidates' mental health problems: a scoping review. *Higher Education Research and Development* 38 (3): 565–578.

22. Kingswell, C., Shaban, R.Z., and Crilly, J. (2015). The lived experiences of patients and ambulance ramping in a regional Australian emergency department: an interpretive phenomenology study. *Australasian Emergency Nursing Journal* 18 (4): 182–189.

23. O'Meara, P. (2015). Searching for paramedic academics: vital for our future, but nowhere to be seen! *Australasian Journal of Paramedicine* 4 (4): 990228.

Section 2

Career Stages and Case Study Exemplars

Chapter 4

Novice Researcher

Elisha Miller

Yorkshire Ambulance Service
NHS Trust, Yorkshire Ambulance
Service Research Institute,
Wakefield, West Yorkshire, England,
United Kingdom

Chapter Objectives

1. Define 'novice researcher' in the context of paramedic practice.
2. Describe the steps of integrating research into paramedic practice.

Research-focused Careers for Paramedics, First Edition.
Edited by Gregory A. Whitley and Scott Munro.
© 2025 John Wiley & Sons Ltd. Published 2025 by John Wiley & Sons Ltd.

3. Discuss research participation using case study exemplars.
4. Discuss research delivery using case study exemplars.
5. Highlight rewards and challenges of this career stage from a paramedic novice researcher perspective.
6. Explore case studies written by paramedics working as novice researchers who describe their research journey and motivators for pursuing a research-focused career.

Beginning a Career as a Novice Paramedic Researcher

Paramedics play a critical role in the healthcare system, providing essential pre-hospital care in emergency situations. While the practical and immediate nature of their work is well recognised, the importance of their involvement in research is often underestimated.

The primary goal of any healthcare profession is to improve patient outcomes, with research being a fundamental tool in achieving this goal. Research in paramedicine plays a critical role in developing evidence-based practice, improving patient outcomes, and shaping healthcare policy. Engaging in research allows paramedics to:

- *Contribute to the body of knowledge*: By conducting research, paramedics can add to the existing literature, helping to refine and improve healthcare practices.
- *Improve patient care*: Research findings can lead to better clinical guidelines, protocols, and interventions, directly impacting the quality of care provided to patients.
- *Develop professional skills*: Engaging in research hones critical thinking skills and enhances one's understanding of medical science.

Researchers at the early stage of their career are defined as novice researchers—which is defined as those entering the research field with little or no experience or any previous publications [1]. Novice researchers typically have limited experience in designing, conducting, and analysing research studies and will usually require substantial guidance and mentorship from more experienced researchers. They may have a working understanding of the various stages of the research process through completion of their university dissertation or research proposal but will generally lack detailed knowledge in relation to study design and the required ethical approvals. Novice researchers are typically at the pre-bachelor's, bachelor's, or master's level of academic training.

> *"I realised during one of my units that emergency research is often completed in the emergency departments in hospital and that there is a huge scope for more relevant research to be done for paramedicine by paramedics."*
>
> Case Study 3

Paramedics who are at the novice researcher stage may have *participated* in some research activities, such as assisting with patient recruitment or data collection whilst working as a recruiting ambulance paramedic, or they may volunteer their time and participate in research studies as a participant, by completing surveys, or being interviewed as part of a qualitative research study, for example. They may have *delivered* research whilst working as part of a research team or department, under the role of a 'research paramedic', for example. These roles typically involve

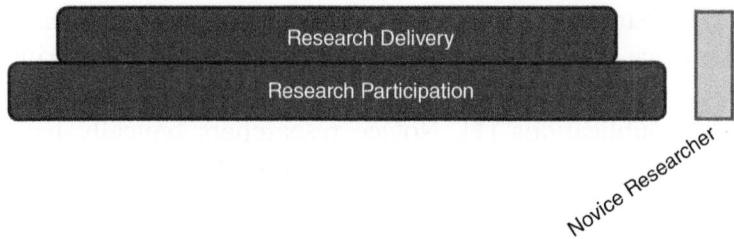

Figure 4.1   Novice Researcher

advertising research studies across organisations, recruiting staff, delivering any necessary training, collecting data, and following up patients who have been recruited. See **Figure 4.1**.

Alongside clinical practice, leadership and management, and education, research and development (R&D) is one of the four pillars of advanced practice and is a segment of the College of Paramedics Career Framework [2]. Within a research-focused career, research participation and delivery are fundamental aspects, and as such, paramedics are expected to have an understanding of research processes and participate in clinical research to ensure they are providing relevant evidence-based practice.

> *"I realised the potential to contribute to the field of paramedicine on a larger scale through research. Noticing the same authors' names repeatedly in journals, I wanted to lift those names off the page and connect with the real people behind them, aspiring to meet, discuss, interact, and ultimately join them in advancing pre-hospital research."*
>
> Case Study 2

Paramedics Participating in Research

Paramedics are on the front line of emergency medical services, providing critical care in dynamic and often challenging environments. While their primary focus is on immediate patient care, their involvement in research is equally vital when considering advancing pre-hospital care research as they are uniquely positioned to contribute to clinical research and trials. As a result, the pre-hospital arena is now witnessing changes to the paramedic role with clinicians now taking on the role of researchers.

As much of the historical clinical literature has been hospital based, documents and policies were created in an effort to understand the barriers to pre-hospital research alongside promotion of the ambulance service as a suitable participant of clinical research. Aiming to enhance pre-hospital research in the UK, the National Institute for Health and Care Research (NIHR) published its findings from the 'Care at the Scene: Research for Ambulance Services' [3] document, which identified several barriers to paramedic participation in research, notably the challenges of managing critically ill patients in a high-pressure environment, limited time, and concerns about professional autonomy.

Recognising the need for enhanced research within allied health professions, Health Education England developed the Allied Health Professions' Research and Innovation Strategy for England [4]. This strategy outlined four key domains for fostering research growth:

- *Empowering the workforce*: building capacity and active engagement in research
- *Developing research skills*: equipping individuals with the necessary capabilities to conduct research

- *Equal access to support*: ensuring equitable access to resources and investment
- *Cultivating a research-inclusive culture*: promoting a climate where research is considered accessible and beneficial for all

These domains for fostering research growth developed by Health Education England are widely applicable to the international paramedicine community and are embedded in grass-roots paramedic research capacity development projects such as the McNally Project based in Canada. The pathway towards a research career is often unclear, with many paramedics simply unsure how to get started, hence the need for initiatives such as the McNally Project.

> *"I can think of two challenges. This first was the difficulty in getting started in research. I knew where I wanted to go, but I had no idea how to get there. Engaging with my university's research department and within my ambulance trust provided the support and guidance needed on CPD and university modules and gaining research, helping me build a suitable CV."*
>
> Case Study 2

Although there has been a significant growth in high-quality pre-hospital research over the last decade, paramedics having the opportunity to engage in research has historically been difficult for reasons such as lack of employer support, a lack of motivation to participate in research and moral concerns relating to capturing consent [5]. For those novice researchers with a research interest and motivation for involvement, they frequently face obstacles which hinder their research opportunities.

> *"An initial challenge for me was juggling operational work with the completion of my research. I found that I needed to be quite organised with timelines and communication to meet both my operational and project milestones. Once I had a system in place the workloads became quite manageable."*
>
> Case Study 3

These obstacles include internal resistance to conducting clinical research and a lack of clarity regarding the necessary steps from idea generation through to delivery and analysis. Specifically, novice researchers may struggle with [6]:

- Initiating the research process due to being uncertain of how to begin
- Time constraints and balancing research with clinical obligations
- Difficulties with securing financial support for conference or course attendance
- Adequate mentorship due to a lack of guidance and support from experienced researchers or the inability to access appropriate research mentors
- Writing and presentation skills as a result of limited knowledge of how to write an effective research proposal or a paper for publication

> *"I am currently studying for a Master's degree—offering me the opportunity to do my own research for the first time. This is incredibly exciting but not without setback and disappointment! Navigating the various forms and approvals has been difficult and there always seems to be one more step before final approval of my study—of course these are in place to ensure safety and rigour."*
>
> Case Study 4

Where these barriers can be alleviated, for those with a pre-hospital interest in research participation, paramedics can take on various roles in research trials, each role contributing uniquely to the success and integrity of the study.

Paramedic Participation in Clinical Trials

Several notable, large-scale clinical trials have been delivered with a significant contribution from ambulance services and with recruiting paramedics delivering the trial intervention, overcoming significant historical barriers to pre-hospital research. The PARAMEDIC out-of-hospital cardiac arrest trials sponsored by the University of Warwick, UK, are large-scale, multi-site trials examining mechanical versus manual chest compressions in out-of-hospital cardiac arrest (PARAMEDIC) [7], adrenaline versus placebo in out-of-hospital cardiac arrest (PARAMEDIC-2) [8], and a strategy of intravenous vascular access first versus a strategy of intraosseous vascular access first for drug administration in out-of-hospital cardiac arrest (PARAMEDIC-3) [9]. Other large-scale pre-hospital trials include the AIRWAYS-2 trial which compared a strategy of supraglottic airway device first versus a strategy of tracheal intubation first in patients who had experienced out-of-hospital cardiac arrest [10] and the RIGHT-2 trial which examined paramedic applied glyceryl trinitrate transdermal patches versus placebo patches to reduce the blood pressure of patients who were experiencing symptoms of an acute stroke. The ability for paramedics to participate in substantial pre-hospital, randomised controlled trials highlights the progression that the paramedic profession has undergone from the provision of simple first aid to registered, autonomous clinicians with a significant understanding of both clinical and research processes.

> *"Research paramedics trained me to participate in the PARAMEDIC-2 and PRESTO studies—enrolling eligible patients that I attended as a 'normal' ambulance paramedic. The reasons behind the studies and their potential impacts fascinated me and I saw research as the opportunity to ask 'why?'."*
>
> Case Study 4

Paramedic participation within these trials requires undergoing trial-specific training in ethical considerations such as the Declaration of Helsinki and Good Clinical Practice (GCP) guidelines and trial protocol adherence to be able to identify and recruit eligible participants. As paramedics are the first healthcare professional at the scene of an emergency call, they are well suited to identify and recruit eligible participants for research trials.

Whilst working in the role of a recruiting paramedic, clinicians are expected to obtain consent, assent, or defer consent, collect vital baseline data at the scene, such as patient demographics, clinical observations and instances of adverse events or symptoms, whilst also carrying out detailed documentation of any treatments administered, including the research intervention. Paramedics must maintain accurate and thorough records to support the research findings as these data are crucial for understanding the context and outcome of the trial whilst reporting any adverse events or complications as this is crucial to ensure patient safety and trial integrity.

Paramedic Participation in Other Research

Although much paramedic research participation is in the form of large-scale clinical trials which evaluate the efficacy of new medications or treatments, paramedics can also participate in a wide range of other research trials such as medical device trials for patients presenting with a specific condition [11] or public health and community-based research such as vaccine trials or health education programmes which aim to improve public health outcomes [12, 13].

Participation can be as simple as helping another researcher with screening articles with an evidence review:

> *"I started with article screening for other honours students."*
> Case Study 3

Paramedics may participate in surveys, qualitative interviews, or focus group studies by providing their time and opinions on certain topics. They may be involved in consensus methods where they either vote on and prioritise items or work towards an agreed definition.

Paramedics play a crucial role in advancing pre-hospital care through participation in research studies. Through this engagement, not only can paramedics enhance their clinical practice, contribute to the evidence-base, and drive improvements in patient outcomes but participation also provides an opportunity to develop future clinical–academic research skills and experience, making it an essential component of the evolution of emergency medical services.

> *"My current plan is to work operationally and find a subject that I would eventually like to turn into a PhD project. I hope to contribute to other projects as a participant or research assistant in the meantime."*
>
> Case Study 3

Paramedics Delivering Research

Research delivery is a fundamental component of the study process, ensuring that research is executed effectively and efficiently from conception to study closure. For paramedics, understanding research delivery is crucial to contributing meaningfully to pre-hospital clinical studies and improving patient care.

Once a study has undergone funding acquisition, received the required ethical approvals and all study processes have been formally confirmed, research delivery can then occur. Ambulance services take a finalised study protocol and create innovative ways of delivering the research across their Trust, utilising their own individual methods and operating procedures (within the scope of the protocol) to ensure that the study is delivered successfully.

The research paramedic role, designed to blend theory and practice, is a role with a specific appeal to those with a research interest where the predominant tasks are to support, promote, and deliver pre-hospital research [14]. The tasks and responsibilities of a research paramedic can vary dependent upon the specific research project being undertaken, but generally encompass:

- Study advertisement
- The creation of trial-specific policies, patient group directions, or standard operating procedures where required
- Delivering training of the protocol to recruiting paramedics or deliverance of the study if it is research paramedic led
- Follow-up of trial participants
- Reporting of adverse or serious events, alongside data collection, analysis, and input

Other responsibilities include but are not limited to engaging with stakeholders or research partners to build a relationship for future collaborations and promote ambulance service research, presenting research both internally and externally at conferences and seminars to disseminate knowledge to the wider community, and writing study results for publication in peer-reviewed journals [15].

Within ambulance services, many of these tasks are carried out by research paramedics working within a R&D team, with potential variances in models of research delivery between United Kingdom and overseas R&D teams.

Research delivery often requires troubleshooting and managing challenges, such as low participant recruitment rates.

"I worked on the delivery of a study surveying paramedics on current practice around end-of-life patients. The team were aware we have been struggling for paramedic participation recently due to increased service pressure, industrial action and other factors so had low expectations for recruitment. I found an opportunity to be involved in face-to-face CPD [continuing professional development] days specific to end of life care. These were well attended by engaged clinicians which enabled great opportunity to promote the study by doing a short presentation. It was well received and as a result the study recruited higher than expected at our site."

Case Study 1

Novice paramedics who wish to progress their clinical academic career may also be in a position to apply for grants and funding to design and deliver independent research with the support of their host organisation. Funding organisations such as professional bodies, charities, government grants, and institutional awards are suitable avenues for novice researchers to apply for funding to design and deliver an independent research project with the potential for future progression through to larger funding streams once more experience has been gained.

Effective research delivery can improve patient care through the generation of robust study data which may underpin future evidence-based practice and policy changes by providing the justification for new interventions that may contribute to the advancement of paramedic-led care. Research delivery also allows novice researchers to develop their understanding of research through mentorship from senior researchers, exposure to training and development opportunities to enhance their research knowledge as well as occasions to network and collaborate with other researchers.

> *"Research is about people. Contact and networking with the incredible people in the field has guided me on my journey. I have found people at all levels are engaged and love to talk about their research with passion and enthusiasm."*
>
> Case Study 2

Due simply to the nature of their clinical role, paramedics are ideally placed to deliver high-quality research that can contribute to evidence-based practice and ultimately improve patient outcomes.

Bridging Academia and Practice—Bachelor's- and Master's-Level Education

As paramedicine continues to evolve, the role of a paramedic is also evolving beyond what was historically simple first aid provision and hospital transportation to the clinically driven emergency ambulance services we know today. As a result, paramedicine now includes the autonomous utilisation of advanced clinical interventions, an improved paramedic drug formulary, the ability to carry out an enhanced and thorough patient assessment, student mentorship, and participation in clinical research.

The expansion of the paramedic role has been driven by the necessity to improve pre-hospital care and the utilisation of evidence-based practice to ensure compliance with modern day contemporary medicine. Historically, paramedic training courses were carried out 'in house' with notable differences in training between geographical areas and the nature of the training that was offered. Training was generally focused on practical skills and the application of clinical interventions, with research not typically being a fundamental aspect of their training and development.

Bachelor's-Level Education

Many countries have now moved to a full bachelor's degree with honours as the minimum requirement for professional registration as a paramedic, including the United Kingdom, Ireland, and Australia. This enhanced programme of education allows for important learning around research and evidence-based practice in the form of a dissertation or research proposal. With more paramedics graduating with a bachelor's degree and progressing quickly onto master's degrees, more pre-hospital research roles such as research paramedics and research fellows are being introduced by ambulance services [5].

The College of Paramedics UK [2] and the Paramedic Association of Canada [16] have produced career framework models that guide the development of paramedics along the research trajectory. Both models proposed the entry level when pursuing a career in research as a 'research paramedic', which aligns to bachelor's level of education with honours. At this level, Griffiths and

Mooney [17] state that those working as research paramedics should be able to carry out simple research tasks such as an evaluation of research techniques and procedures, undertake simple audits, assist with clinical trials and projects, and undertake research projects.

With bachelor's-level education, paramedics have the ability to participate in the evolution of research and drive their progression due to their enhanced knowledge and skills, enabling them to implement study protocols and deliver high-quality research. When considering bachelor's-level university courses, the primary aim is to enhance the critical thinking and independent practice of paramedics, equipping them with the confidence and readiness to transition into proficient clinicians and ensure their preparedness for the expanded responsibilities and roles that they can assume within research.

While a clear career path for paramedics interested in research is slowly improving with the introduction of various paramedic career frameworks, a bachelor's degree can provide paramedic novice researchers with a valuable foundation. These undergraduate programmes often emphasise evidence-based practice and introduce students to research methodologies, offering a crucial steppingstone into future research-related roles, highlighting the benefits of a university accredited BSc qualification [15]. Despite this, the entire research process, comprising of research study design, delivery, and subsequent publication, can be challenging for novice bachelor's-level researchers to implement due to their lack of prior experience. To address this challenge, universities offer research training at master's level.

> *"Although things are changing, in my experience as a paramedic we like to point out things that could be different but rarely do anything about it. By investing in a culture of evidence-based practice and thinking, we can improve our working life, our own health, patient outcomes, and the impact that has on their friends and family. By knowing what doesn't work, what does work and what works even better, we can keep improving."*
>
> Case Study 4

Master's-Level Education

Relevant research master's degrees include Master's by Research (MRes), Master's in Clinical Research (MClinRes), Master of Science (MSc) degree, or other (see **Chapter 3, Education**). These postgraduate degrees require the completion of a research project, they provide researchers with an understanding of research methodologies and will equip aspiring PhD students with the necessary skills and knowledge to pursue future doctoral research. Varying by university, the common teaching aspects of a postgraduate degree include research techniques alongside several other transferable skills such as presenting skills, report writing, communication, data management, project preparation, statistical methods, and experimental design [18]. The degree will emphasise the importance of research by teaching paramedics how to design and deliver research and analyse any generated results, whilst providing opportunities to develop critical thinking skills and evidence-based practice.

Upon completion of a postgraduate master's degree, the College of Paramedics UK framework postulates that paramedics should be working at the Research Fellow/Senior Research Paramedic level which involves being at the forefront of innovation in paramedicine and driving the development and implementation of evidence-based practice through leading on original research projects. The Paramedic Association of Canada offer guidance, stating that paramedics with a master's degree may work at the level of:

- *Research fellow*: advanced knowledge with the ability to conduct research studies, synthesise findings, and inform organisational processes
- *Scientist*: senior research leadership with responsibility for a portfolio of research programs and staff, ability to inform policy and processes

Paramedic Association of Canada [16].

Whilst the term 'research fellow' is typically associated with postdoctoral researchers with significant research experience based at higher education institutions, within the ambulance service the title may be used for paramedic researchers who do not have a doctoral qualification but have moderate research experience coupled with extensive clinical experience. Academic qualifications do not always align to levels of career development and doctoral qualifications are not required to become an expert researcher, a core example being Emeritus Professor Tom Quinn, MPhil, who has made a profound impact in the fields of cardiovascular and pre-hospital research.

When considering the progression of pre-hospital research, an aspect of the research fellow/senior research paramedic/scientist role is the identification of research opportunities through comprehensive literature searches with the target being to secure funding opportunities for future research studies. Paramedics at this postgraduate level are also expected to take the lead when carrying out systematic or literature reviews and the publication of research outputs in peer-reviewed journals.

Starting with manageable, small-scale research projects at the bachelor's level can build confidence and experience. Once paramedics progress through to the postgraduate level, they are able to independently identify and develop research opportunities that generate a wider external impact [17]. It is important to remember that research projects do not have to carry a clinical focus, they may focus on professional development, education, leadership, even the environment:

> "I am passionate about the environment and see NHS net-zero targets in 2050 as something to be achieved in my career. I'd like to be a key contributor in building the evidence base for changes that help achieve this."
>
> Case Study 1

Postgraduate paramedic novice researchers play a crucial role in expanding pre-hospital research, and through leading research initiatives, research fellows are instrumental in advancing knowledge and evidence-based practice that can benefit not only pre-hospital clinicians but the wider population also.

Research participation is becoming increasingly accessible due to the increasing number of pre-hospital trials being offered within ambulance services, with opportunities for participation at each stage from initial idea creation, through to research delivery and subsequent publication, with paramedics being in a prime position to identify areas requiring improvement and deliver high-quality research.

> *"I've often been told, don't be downhearted following a rejection—be it funding, publication or something else, it's part and parcel of a career in research. Take onboard feedback and learn for next time."*
>
> Case Study 1

Chapter Summary

Paramedics have a vital role to play in advancing the field of pre-hospital care through research. Through this engagement, paramedics can enhance patient care, advance their professional development, and contribute to the knowledge that shapes the future of pre-hospital research. Despite the challenges, the benefits of paramedic involvement in research are profound, making it an essential aspect of a modern, evidence-based approach to pre-hospital care. By understanding the importance of research and taking active steps to engage in it, paramedics can not only improve their practice but also make meaningful contributions to the broader healthcare community.

Becoming a competent researcher is a journey that involves continuous learning and development. As a novice researcher, embracing opportunities for education, mentorship, and practical experience will lay a strong foundation for a successful research career. Patience, perseverance, and a willingness to learn from both successes and setbacks are key to progressing from novice to expert in the field of research.

Case Studies in Paramedic Research

Four paramedic novice researchers, with differing starts to their research journey, have provided a case study offering a detailed insight into the real world of pre-hospital research. They discuss their motivators for pursuing a research career, any challenges they have encountered, their future career plans or aspirations, alongside top tips to assist other novice researchers in forging their own career pathway.

Case Study 1

Name: Mr Alex Diffley

Job title: Research Paramedic

Affiliation(s): Yorkshire Ambulance Service NHS Trust, West Yorkshire Health and Care Partnership.

Short biography of your career.
I started as an operational paramedic in 2017 having completed my DipHE at Sheffield Hallam University. Early on I trained as a recruiting paramedic in the RIGHT-2 trial. In 2018, I started a top-up degree at Bradford University where I particularly enjoyed critical appraisal. In 2020, I successfully applied to join my trust's quality improvement (QI) fellowship, a secondment to learn and then implement QI methodologies to small-scale improvements. Given the COVID-19 pandemic, this

(continued)

(continued)

was delayed until 2021. This opened my eyes to the bigger picture of how the ambulance service works and where gaps in knowledge, data, or evidence existed. I joined my trusts research and development (R&D) team in September 2021. I worked mostly in research delivery. In 2022, I started a National Institute for Health and Care Research (NIHR)-funded master's program in Leading Research Delivery, firstly at Newcastle University (PGCert), moving to Exeter University (MSc) in 2023. I am now working towards developing my own research alongside continuing in research delivery and governance.

Key motivators for pursuing a research career.
I am passionate about the environment and see NHS net-zero targets in 2050 as something to be achieved in my career. I'd like to be a key contributor in building the evidence base for changes that help achieve this.

A specific challenge you have faced pursuing and undertaking this stage of your career.
I spotted, what I felt, was a flaw in some documentation for a study I was helping deliver. I am still early in my research career, so often find myself suffering a touch of imposter syndrome, 'I'm just a paramedic, I don't know as much as these experienced clinical trials units (CTUs), higher education institutions (HEIs), etc.' But I am growing in expertise, particularly in delivering research in the ambulance sector—which is different to delivery in hospital. I am growing in confidence and learning when my expertise is needed. In this case I was right, I advised the

chief investigators (CIs) who adjusted the documentation to aid training in this study.

Benefits/rewards of pursuing a career in research.
I worked on the delivery of a study surveying paramedics on current practice around end-of-life patients. The team were aware we have been struggling for paramedic participation recently due to increased service pressure, industrial action and other factors, so had low expectations for recruitment. I found an opportunity to be involved in face-to-face continuing professional development (CPD) days specific to end-of-life care. These were well attended by engaged clinicians which enabled great opportunity to promote the study by doing a short presentation. It was well received and as a result the study recruited higher than expected at our site.

Future plans and top tips/advice to others considering a career in research.
My next big goals are to be a lead author on a publication and gain continuing funding for my master's. I've often been told, don't be downhearted following a rejection—be it funding, publication, or something else, it's part and parcel of a career in research. Take onboard feedback and learn for next time. My main advice would be to embrace the power of networking. Go to conferences, talk to people, there are so many researchers and clinicians happy to share their knowledge and I certainly seem to bump into people who can help my work, likely because we go to similar events.

Case Study 2

Name: Mr Andy Cole

Job title: Lead Research Paramedic

Affiliation(s): South Western Ambulance Service NHS Foundation Trust

Short biography of your career.
I joined the ambulance service five years ago as an emergency care assistant (ECA) with aspirations of becoming a paramedic. During my studies I developed a renewed interest in research, having previously completed an MSc in sports injury rehabilitation. This background paved the way for opportunities I have enjoyed while working for my Trust.

Currently, I am an newly qualified paramedic (NQP) and didn't expect any opportunities in research to arise before completing this period. However, I engaged in several research projects during this time and applied for a research paramedic role when another research paramedic posted the job in one of our research project WhatsApp groups.

Fortunately, I was successful in securing an interview and subsequently a role in the research team for which I am very grateful. I am currently completing level 7 modules funded by my Trust, including one in research methodology. In my new role, I am working on the cardiac arrest registry, a very important and worthwhile endeavour.

Key motivators for pursuing a research career.
During my paramedic course, I realised the potential to contribute to the field of paramedicine on a larger scale

through research. Noticing the same authors' names repeatedly in journals, I wanted to lift those names off the page and connect with the real people behind them, aspiring to meet, discuss, interact, and ultimately join them in advancing pre-hospital research.

A specific challenge you have faced pursuing and undertaking this stage of your career.
I can think of two challenges. This first was the difficulty in getting started in research. I knew where I wanted to go, but I had no idea how to get there. Engaging with my university's research department and within my ambulance trust provided the support and guidance needed on CPD and university modules and gaining research, helping me build a suitable CV.

Secondly, in my research paramedic role, cleansing data for the cardiac arrest registry to the appropriate standard took several months. I used feedback from colleagues to build my own logic check sheet ensuring data quality and accuracy.

Benefits/rewards of pursuing a career in research.
I am still new to research and relish learning something new every day. I feel privileged to contribute to the national cardiac arrest registry, and tackling the other challenges it presents, such as providing data for all sorts of questions and queries and steering guidelines. It is humbling to see how many individuals within our trust manage the most serious events in patient's lives from a vast perspective not seen in day-to-day practice. Recently I have completed a research proposal involving the registry, which

(continued)

(continued)

I hope can contribute to the growing body of evidence in cardiac arrest research.

Future plans and top tips/advice to others considering a career in research.
What most excites me about research is the endless journey it offers. I hope to continue my MSc studies and pursue a PhD program if the opportunity arises. If that doesn't happen, I look forward to seeing where the research takes me!

My advice is that research is about people. Contact and networking with the incredible people in the field has guided me on my journey. I have found people at all levels are engaged and love to talk about their research with passion and enthusiasm. Additionally, volunteer and offer to contribute in any way you can, then you can be part of something much bigger than yourself.

Case Study 3

Name: Miss Hannah Lindsay

Job title: Ambulance Paramedic

Affiliation(s): Ambulance Victoria, Monash University

Short biography of your career.
I am a rural ambulance paramedic in my second year operational, having recently finished my graduate program. Prior to this I completed three years of undergraduate university and chose to continue into the honours

program as a fourth and fifth year. I started with article screening for other honours students. Towards the end of my degree, I became increasingly interested in the topic of airways. I brought this interest to a Senior Lecturer that I highly regarded and asked for his advice as to how I could research and contribute to the subject. He took me on and became a mentor for my project, as well as bringing on another subject matter expert to be my second mentor. A key moment for me was attending and presenting my research at an international conference. It felt amazing to share what I found interesting and learn from others what their research passions were.

Key motivators for pursuing a research career.
I had some exposure to research throughout university. I realised during one of my units that emergency research is often completed in the emergency departments in hospital and that there is a huge scope for more relevant research to be done for paramedicine by paramedics.

A specific challenge you have faced pursuing and undertaking this stage of you career.
An initial challenge for me was juggling operational work with the completion of my research. I found that I needed to be quite organised with timelines and communication to meet both my operational and project milestones. Once I had a system in place the workloads became quite manageable. I completed an experimental study design, which required equipment, volunteers, and real-time data collection. At first, this seemed like a very large task; however, I had an incredibly supportive team of mentors

(continued)

(continued)

behind me who were more than happy to set an example for how the experimental days might run, and answer any questions or concerns that I had.

Benefits/rewards of pursuing a career in research. I found that attending conferences and even being able to present at one was wonderful. Being surrounded by like-minded people who are interested in research and sharing their knowledge is very rewarding and only increased my interest in being a researcher. Paramedicine is also uniquely young. I feel like there is so much to contribute to the field and it was very satisfying knowing that even though my project was small, it can add to the body of evidence and still make a difference to operations. Using the equipment at work that I was concurrently investigating in my project was surreal and satisfying.

Future plans and top tips/advice to others considering a career in research. I don't think I will ever stop being curious and asking questions. My current plan is to work operationally and find a subject that I would eventually like to turn into a PhD project. I hope to contribute to other projects as a participant or research assistant in the meantime. My advice would be to let yourself become involved in the community of academics and ask for help if you need it! You're not alone and you're probably not going to reinvent the wheel which is okay! Build a network of experienced academics that you can ask for help but don't forget the novices that are in the same boat as you!

Case Study 4

Name: Mr Owen Stanley

Job title: Research Paramedic

Affiliation(s): West Midlands Ambulance Service University NHS Foundation Trust

Short biography of your career.
I joined the ambulance service straight after A-levels so constant learning was still a big part of me. After qualifying as a paramedic, what I was learning each day wasn't very obvious and I needed to know more. I'm a curious person and being taught based on expert opinion of years gone by with no question just wasn't in me. I am now a research paramedic that gets to ask questions every day and help shape the future of my profession and the care we can offer patients and ourselves in a modern, ever-changing world.

Key motivators for pursuing a research career.
Research paramedics trained me to participate in the PARAMEDIC-2 and PRESTO studies—enrolling eligible patients that I attended as a 'normal' ambulance paramedic. The reasons behind the studies and their potential impacts fascinated me and I saw research as the opportunity to ask 'why?'.

A specific challenge you have faced pursuing and undertaking this stage of you career.
I am currently studying for a master's degree—offering me the opportunity to do my own research for the first

(continued)

(continued)

time. This is incredibly exciting but not without setback and disappointment! Navigating the various forms and approvals has been difficult and there always seems to be one more step before final approval of my study—of course these are in place to ensure safety and rigour.

Seeking advice from those with experience seems the best approach, each study requires different approval pathways and documentation so there isn't a simple flow-chart to follow. Experienced peers (and those reading the forms and granting approval) seem more than happy to help new researchers.

Benefits/rewards of pursuing a career in research.
My role is more varied than ever; working with patients, paramedics, other ambulance service staff, universities, and big datasets. I explain to paramedics why they should care about research and enable them to participate them-selves. I sit with patients and talk them carefully through a study they were involved in and follow up to see how our care has affected them. I help develop new studies, deliver them, and report findings.

For me, having my own study approved gives me the confidence that I know how and why research is done to provide the most useful outcome for those affected, be that patients or clinicians.

Future plans and top tips/advice to others considering a career in research.
Never stop asking. Everything we do (or don't do!) as par-amedics is for a reason. We don't always know that reason or agree with the reason and that's where I see research at it's prime.

Although things are changing, in my experience as a paramedic we like to point out things that could be different but rarely do anything about it. By investing in a culture of evidence-based practice and thinking, we can improve our working life, our own health, patient outcomes, and the impact that has on their friends and family.

By knowing what doesn't work, what does work, and what works even better, we can keep improving.

References

1. Jatin, S., Anand, S. & Ricardo, P. Scientific writing of novice researchers: what difficulties and encouragements do they encounter? *Academic Medicine* (2018). 84(4): 511–516. doi:https://doi.org/10.1097/ACM.0b013e31819a8c3c.

2. College of Paramedics (2024). Paramedic career framework 2022 5th edition revised. https://collegeofparamedics.co.uk/COP/ProfessionalDevelopment/post_reg_career_framework.aspx (accessed 19 December 2023).

3. National Institute for Health and Care Research (2016). Care at the scene: research for ambulance services. https://aace.org.uk/wp-content/uploads/2016/05/Care-at-the-scene-final-for-web.pdf (accessed 04 March 2024).

4. Health Education England (2022). Allied health professions research and innovation strategy for England. https://www.hee.nhs.uk/sites/default/files/documents/HEE%20Allied%20Health%20Professions%20Research%20and%20Innovation%20Strategy%20FINAL_0.pd (accessed 04 March 2024).

5. Runacres, J., Harvey, H., O'brien, S., and Halck, A. (2024). Paramedics as researchers: a systematic review of paramedic perspectives of engaging in research activity from training to practice. *The Journal of Emergency Medicine* 66 (6): 680–689. https://doi.org/10.1016/j.jemermed.2024.01.008.

6. Tago, M., Hirata, R., Shikino, K., Watari, T., Sasaki, Y., Takahashi, H. & Shimizu, T. The milestones of clinical research for young

generalist physicians: conducting and publishing studies. *International Journal of General Medicine* (2023). 16: 2373–2381. doi:https://doi.org/10.2147/IJGM.S411687.

7. Perkins, G., Lall, R., Quinn, T. et al. (2015). Mechanical versus manual chest compression for out-of-hospital cardiac arrest (PARAMEDIC): a pragmatic, cluster randomised controlled trial. *The Lancet* 385: 947–955. https://doi.org/10.1016/S0140-6736(14)61886-9.

8. Perkins, G., Ji, C., Deakin, C., Quinn, T., Nolan, J., Scomparin, C., Regan, S., Long, J., Slowther, A., Pocock, H., Black, J., Moore, F., Fothergill, R., Rees, N., O'Shea, L., Docherty, M., Gunson, I., Han, K., Charlton, K., Finn, J., Petrou, S., Stallard, N., Gates, S. & Lall, R. A randomised trial of epinephrine in out-of-hospital cardiac arrest. *The New England Journal of Medicine* (2018). 379(8):711–721.doi:https://doi.org/10.1056/NEJMoa1806842.

9. Couper, K., Ji, C., Lall, R., Deakin, C., Fothergill, R., Long, J., Mason, J., Michelet, F., Nolan, J., Nwankwo, H., Quinn, T., Slowther, A., Smyth, M., Walker, A., Chowdhury, L., Norman, C., Sprauve, L., Starr, K., Wood, S., Bell, S., Bradley, G., Brown, M., Brown, S., Charlton, K., Coppola, A., Evans, C., Evans, C., Foster, T., Jackson, M., Kearney, J., Lang, N., Mellett-Smith, A., Osborne, R., Pocock, H., Rees, N., Spaight, R., Tibbetts, B., Whitley, G., Wiles, J., Williams, J., Wright, A. & Perkins, G. Route of drug administration in out-of-hospital cardiac arrest: a protocol for a randomised controlled trial (PARAMEDIC-3). *Resuscitation Plus.* (2024). 17. doi:https://doi.org/10.1016/j.resplu.2023.100544.

10. Benger, J., Kirby, K., Black, S., Brett, S., Clout, M., Lazaroo, M., Nolan, J., Reeves, B., Robinson, M., Scott, L., Smartt, H., South, A., Stokes, E., Taylor, J., Thomas, M., Voss, S., Wordsworth, S. & Rogers, C. Effect of a strategy of a supraglottic airway device vs tracheal intubation during out-of-hospital cardiac arrest on functional outcome: the AIRWAYS-2 randomised controlled trial. *JAMA* (2018). 320 (8): 779–791. doi:https://doi.org/10.1001/jama.2018.11597.

11. University of Exeter (2023). Ambulance service trials new device for patients with fast heartbeat. https://news.exeter.ac.uk/faculty-of-health-and-life-sciences/ambulance-service-trials-new-device-for-patients-with-fast-heartbeat/ (accessed 03 January 2024).

12. Marincowitz, C., Sutton, L., Stone, T., Pilbery, R., Campbell, R., Thomas, B., Turner, J., Bath, P., Bell, F., Biggs, K., Hasan, M., Hopfgartner, F., Mazumdar, S., Petrie, J. & Goodacre, S. Prognostic accuracy of triage tools for adults with suspected COVID-19 in a prehospital setting: an observational cohort study. *Emergency Medicine Journal* (2022). 39 (4):317–324. doi:https://doi.org/10.1136/emermed-2021-211934.

13. Ablard, S., Miller, E., Poulton, S. et al. (2023). Delivery of public health interventions by the ambulance sector: a scoping review. *BMC Public Health* 23 (1): https://doi.org/10.1186/s12889-023-16473-2.

14. McClelland, G., Limmer, M., and Charlton, K. (2023). The RESearch PARamedic Experience (RESPARE) study: a qualitative study exploring the experiences of research paramedics working in the United Kingdom. *British Paramedic Journal* 7 (4): 14–22. https://doi.org/10.29045/14784726.2023.3.7.4.14.

15. McClelland, G. (2013). The research paramedic: a new role. *Journal of Paramedic Practice* 5 (10): 582–586. https://doi.org/10.12968/jpar.2013.5.10.582.

16. Paramedic Association of Canada (2024). PAC career framework for paramedics. https://doi.org/10.17605/OSF.IO/WDH9M (accessed 16 July 2024).

17. Griffiths, P. and Mooney, G. (2012). Research and the paramedic. In: *The Paramedic's Guide to Research: An Introduction* (ed. P. Griffiths and G. Mooney), 1–10. Berkshire: Open University Press.

18. Green, H., Shaw, M., and Hammill, F. (2001). W(h)ither the MRes? *Quality Assurance on Education* 9 (4): 178–183. https://doi.org/10.1108/09684880110408184.

Further Reading

National Institute for Health and Care Research. *Care at the Scene: Research for Ambulance Services* (2016) DOI: https://doi.org/10.3310/themedreview-000827 (accessed 05 August 2024)

NHS England. *Allied Health Professions' Research and Innovation Strategy for England* (2022) https://www.hee.nhs.uk/our-work/allied-health-professions/enable-workforce/allied-health-professions%E2%80%99-research-innovation-strategy-england (accessed 05 August 2024)

College of Paramedics. *Paramedic Career Framework* (2024) https://collegeofparamedics.co.uk/COP/Professional Development/post_reg_career_framework.aspx (accessed 05 August 2024)

College of Paramedics. *Paramedic Post Graduate Career Guidance* (2023) https://collegeofparamedics.co.uk/COP/ProfessionalDevelopment/Post_Graduate_Curriculum_Guidance.aspx (accessed 05 August 2024)

Paramedic Association of Canada. *Career Framework.* (2024) https://paramedic.ca/documents/NCFP/2024%20PAC%20Career%20Framework%20for%20Paramedics%201e.pdf (accessed 05 August 2024)

Siriwardena, A.N. and Whitley, G.A. (2022). *Prehospital Research Methods and Practice.* Bridgwater: Class Professional Publishing ISBN-13: 9781859599808.

Department of Health and Social Care. *Saving and Improving Lives: The Future of UK Clinical Research Delivery* (2021) https://www.gov.uk/governent/publications/the-future-of-uk-clinical-research-delivery/saving-and-improving-lives-the-future-of-uk-clinical-research-delivery (accessed 05 August 2024)

McNally Project (2025) http://mcnallyproject.ca/ (accessed 05 August 2024)

Chapter 5
Competent Researcher

Georgette Eaton[1,2]

[1] London Ambulance Service NHS Trust, London, UK
[2] Nuffield Department of Primary Care Health Sciences, University of Oxford, Oxford, UK

Chapter Objectives

1. Define what it means to be a competent researcher within the field of paramedicine.
2. Explain research design through examples from real-world case studies.
3. Discuss the role of leadership in research projects, using case studies as illustrations.

Research-focused Careers for Paramedics, First Edition.
Edited by Gregory A. Whitley and Scott Munro.
© 2025 John Wiley & Sons Ltd. Published 2025 by John Wiley & Sons Ltd.

Defining a Competent Paramedic Researcher

In a research-oriented career, participation in and delivery of research are essential components. Aspiring paramedic researchers are expected to understand research processes and engage in research to promote research capacity within the profession, and ultimately the delivery of relevant, evidence-based care. From this stage, it is a journey that involves continuous learning and development to become a competent paramedic researcher.

> *"The single lesson which has helped me on this journey is to adopt an explorer mindset. Initially I expected my projects to be clear cut, targeted, and to conform to an exquisitely detailed plan. Research is about problem solving, not 'answer finding.' An answer to a question might be the end product, but that answer is not just lying around waiting for you. Discovering, or constructing it, takes creative thinking, responsiveness, and adaptability as well as tenacity. Researchers need to become comfortable in the unknown, and not be intimidated by uncertainty. If it were not like that it would not be research."*
>
> Case Study 6

A competent researcher also demonstrates strong problem-solving abilities, effective communication skills, and an understanding of ethical guidelines to ensure the integrity and credibility of their work. Additionally, they remain open to new ideas, continuously seek to improve their expertise, and contribute meaningfully to their field.

Paramedics who are at the competent researcher stage will possess the knowledge, skills, and ethical integrity necessary to conduct rigorous, systematic investigations to generate reliable and valid results. Thus, they will be proficient in *research design*. Research design refers to the overall strategy and structure of a research project, outlining how data will be collected, analysed, and interpreted to address the research questions or hypotheses. It serves as a blueprint that guides researchers through the process of conducting the study, ensuring that the methods align with the research objectives and provide valid, reliable, and meaningful results.

A competent researcher also ensures that the project runs smoothly, stays aligned with the research goals, and produces valuable, high-quality outcomes. This encompasses *project leadership*. Project leadership in research refers to the process of guiding, directing, and managing a research project to ensure its successful completion. A project leader in research is responsible for overseeing all aspects of the project, from conceptualisation to execution and dissemination of results, while ensuring that the project stays on track in terms of objectives, timeline, budget, and quality.

However, it's important to acknowledge that research rarely goes exactly to plan, no matter how much preparation is involved. This is not a mark of inexperience, but rather a natural part of the research process. The real skill lies in being flexible, staying resilient, and adapting to the challenges faced. Successful researchers demonstrate their competence by navigating these unexpected difficulties, adjusting their approach when necessary, and still delivering meaningful, impactful outcomes. See **Figure 5.1**.

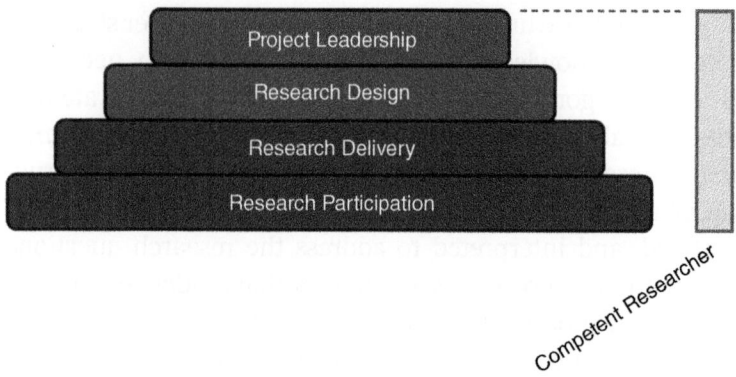

Figure 5.1 Competent Researcher

Paramedics Designing Research

Research design defines the framework and methodology to ensure the research is structured and systematic, leading to credible findings.

Finding the Problem that Needs Addressing Through Research

Identifying a problem that requires research is the foundational step in designing research. This process involves closely observing real-world challenges, gathering input from stakeholders, and analysing gaps in existing knowledge or practice. For example, a paramedic researcher might, through first-hand clinical experience, notice inconsistencies in pain management protocols for children in pre-hospital settings. Recognising this gap, based on their direct involvement in patient care, they identify it as an area requiring further investigation to improve care. This experience-driven insight could lead to a study exploring the safety and effectiveness of alternative pain management strategies, ultimately addressing an important clinical need. By pinpointing specific issues that affect individual patients, communities, systems or a profession, competent researchers can formulate targeted questions that guide their investigations. Addressing these problems through research not only contributes to the academic body of knowledge but also leads to practical solutions that improve outcomes and inform future practices.

"The lack of contextually relevant disciplinary knowledge made solving the clinical and educational problems I was encountering difficult. I applied my newly acquired research skills to the body of literature and produced little. When colleagues and other experts let me know that they too were struggling to find the answers they needed I realised the need for research."

Case Study 6

Learning How to Design Research

For paramedic researchers conducting their first research project, the choice of approach and subsequent alignment among problem, research questions, data collection, and data analysis can be particularly difficult. One of the most substantial hurdles in research design is the knowledge of various approaches to research, and different sets of theoretical frameworks, data collection, and data analysis methods [1].

Formal education for designing research would typically be within master's-level education (see **Chapters 3** and **4**). Whilst there will be variation across different university programmes, postgraduate degrees will typically highlight the significance of research by instructing paramedics on how to cultivate critical thinking skills and evidence-based practice through designing and conducting studies, analysing the results, and appropriate dissemination strategies.

However, for competent researchers, a mixture of formal education and experiences can be fundamental in developing understanding of research design. Informal opportunities for gaining experience in research design and methodology include:

- Fieldwork
  - Gaining experience through hands-on research in real-world settings, typically through research participation and delivery (see **Chapter 4**) can provide practical insights into a range of methodologies.
- Mentorship
  - Seeking out mentors in the field who can help researchers learn about design and methodology through guidance and feedback on their work.

"Mentorship is crucial. Finding a mentor with whom I could hold honest, and sometimes humbling discussions, and with whom I could talk through problems was indispensable. Sometimes an alternate view from someone who understands how you make meaning of things is what is needed. Mentorship was the key for me."

Case Study 6

- Peer review
  - Some journals offer training or mentorship programs in the peer review process, helping researchers refine their ability to critically assess research quality. As well as being a peer reviewer for journals, joining or forming groups to review other's research proposals can foster skill development through constructive criticism.

> *"I looked at high-quality studies that were highlights in the field and looked how experts critiqued them. I then realised that gaining this skill required both a solid foundation in research knowledge and extensive reading in the field. This combination of education and practice significantly improved my ability to evaluate research critically."*
> Case Study 5

- Research communities
  - Joining collaborative teams or networks such as the McNally Project in Canada or the Community for Allied Health Professional Research in the United Kingdom can allow researchers to share ideas and learn from peer's experiences.

> *"I have found inspiration to keep challenging myself (and to keep going) in the research community in paramedicine. I am forced to stretch and grow, and I know I can contribute and have an impact. I have found new friends, colleagues, and collaborators, and have already had additional 'doors opened' because I said yes to pursuing the research arm of my career."*
> Case Study 8

- Workshops or seminars
  - Attending workshops or seminars offered by universities or professional organisations can enhance skills in specific methodologies. Sometimes this training is offered for free, but cost can often be a barrier. However, there may be ways to access funding to support professional development. In some cases, grants are available, and training costs can be included as part of research project funding or fellowships. Additionally, applying for staff development funds from your employer may be an option worth exploring to provide further financial support.

These opportunities can complement formal education and help build a robust skill set in research design and methodology.

Positioning

The Paramedic Association of Canada notes that paramedics who are conducting studies, synthesising findings are typically working as a Research Fellow [2]. This aligns with the UK College of Paramedics career framework [3], where the same titled role would be expected to involve leading original research projects to drive innovation and implement evidence-based practice.

To achieve this, researchers would typically seek employment in settings that supports and encourage research. This is often aligned with universities where the researcher's interests match the institution's research priorities and strategy. Additionally, ambulance and air ambulance services are increasingly employing research fellows, providing further opportunities to conduct meaningful research within pre-hospital care settings.

"It was a tough decision to step away from hands-on patient care, but I realised academia offered a unique platform to improve prehospital care through evidence-based approaches."

Case Study 5

"So, whoever considers a research career need to find a related academic area where research in paramedicine can be carried out."

Case Study 7

Funding

In the United Kingdom, opportunities to develop understanding of research design is supported and encouraged by several key policies and frameworks, particularly from organisations like the National Institute for Health and Care Research (NIHR), which plays a crucial role in driving healthcare research [4]. The NIHR promotes research engagement across healthcare professions, including paramedics, to ensure evidence-based practice and innovation in care. The NIHR offers specific funding programmes which can be used to support paramedics in designing and leading research studies relevant to improving patient outcomes. These programmes are typically aligned to doctoral-level study.

Currently, however, there are fewer such formal-funded opportunities for paramedics outside the United Kingdom—and even within the United Kingdom, such opportunities are highly competitive. Further discussion of funding opportunities for paramedics pursuing a research career can be found in **Chapter 1**. To be a competitive applicant for doctoral funding programs, consider the following advice:

Strong research proposal: Craft a clear, well-structured research proposal that demonstrates originality, relevance, and feasibility. Highlight how your research aligns with current trends or fills a significant gap in the field. Tailor the proposal to the specific priorities of the funding body or university.

Highlight academic and research excellence: Emphasise academic achievements, relevant coursework, and prior research experience. Publications, conference presentations, or research assistant roles add credibility, showing you can produce rigorous work and contribute meaningfully to your field.

Secure strong references: Obtain recommendation letters from professors or mentors who can attest to your research abilities, intellectual curiosity, and commitment. Make sure they can speak specifically to your suitability for a doctoral programme.

Demonstrate alignment with supervisors and programme goals: Research potential supervisors' work and the goals of the program. Demonstrating alignment shows you're a good fit and signals that you'll make the most of their resources.

Showcase soft skills: Highlight skills like critical thinking, perseverance, time management, and collaboration. These are essential in doctoral work, where independence and resilience are required.

Consider additional qualifications: Courses, certifications, or relevant work experience can set you apart, especially if they directly contribute to your research skills or knowledge in the field.

Paramedics Leading Research

Project leadership in research involves guiding and managing a research project from inception to completion. Effective project leadership is crucial for successful research outcomes, as it ensures that projects are executed efficiently and that the team remains focused and motivated.

Defining Objectives and Planning Research

Defining objectives and planning research are essential steps that establish a clear direction for the project, ensuring that specific goals are identified, and a structured approach is developed to guide the research process effectively. This includes outlining methodologies, setting timelines, and allocating resources, all of which help to align the team's efforts and enhance the likelihood of achieving meaningful outcomes.

Team Management

Effective team management, clear communication, and proactive problem-solving are critical components of successful research leadership as a competent researcher. Managing a diverse team involves fostering collaboration and ensuring that each member understands their roles and responsibilities. This may include collaborating with other academics and researchers, staff providing administrative support, patient and public involvement and engagement (PPIE) representatives, finance teams, and human resource teams. Open lines of communication facilitate the sharing of ideas and progress updates, helping to maintain alignment and motivation. Part of team management also requires time management, which for many competent researchers may be how their research is integrated within their life. When challenges arise, a competent researcher uses problem-solving skills to identify issues, explore solutions, and adapt strategies, ensuring that the project stays on track and goals are met.

> *"The greatest challenge is figuring out how to integrate the work into your overall life. Pursuing a PhD part-time, working full time, raising a tiny human, staying physically and mentally healthy, and maintaining capacity to be a compassionate and supportive spouse, parent, colleague, and friend is the biggest challenge. Reflecting on what is important to you, who you are, what your goals are, and learning how to prioritize your needs is the challenging work. It is more about navigating the waters and adjusting as you go versus overcoming the challenge."*
>
> Case Study 8

Ensuring Compliance

Monitoring progress and ensuring compliance are vital for the success of any research project. Regularly assessing milestones and deliverables allows leaders to track the project's trajectory and make timely adjustments as needed. Simultaneously, adhering to ethical standards and institutional guidelines safeguards the integrity of the research. By maintaining oversight on both progress and compliance, competent researchers can ensure that objectives are met while upholding the highest standards of quality and accountability.

> *"As the German ambulance system is organised on a very small scale, the relevant institutions have to be contacted for every piece of research and data collection. In some cases, the medical directors have to be painstakingly persuaded to make the data available."*
>
> Case Study 7

Dissemination

Dissemination is crucial for sharing research findings with a broader audience, as it transforms data and insights into knowledge that can influence practice, policy, and future studies. By effectively communicating results through publications, presentations, and community engagement, researchers ensure that their work reaches relevant stakeholders, including practitioners, policymakers, and the public. This not only enhances the impact of the research but also fosters collaboration and dialogue within the field, ultimately contributing to the advancement of knowledge and improved outcomes in practice. Furthermore, observing the impact on published work and witnessing it influence change can bring a profound sense of personal achievement, as it demonstrates the tangible impact research can have in shaping how things are done and improving patient care.

> *"As a researcher it might be one of the best experiences when you see that your research makes a difference. There were some occasions, were my work or the work carried out by German Society of Paramedic Science (DGRe) colleagues were cited in documents of the German Federal Ministry of Health or in a conference at the parliament—the Bundestag. To see that political decisions with far-reaching consequences are based on the own work is very rewarding."*
>
> Case Study 7

> *"When we finally presented our initial findings, it was incredibly fulfilling. I felt a deep sense of accomplishment knowing that our work could serve as a cornerstone for future studies aimed at improving outcomes for these patients. Being part of developing a national registry felt like a significant contribution to the field, reinforcing my belief in the transformative power of research in healthcare."*
>
> Case Study 5

Inspiring Future Paramedic Researchers

Competent researchers play a vital role in inspiring the next generation of paramedic researchers by modelling best practices, demonstrating the value of evidence-based approaches, and sharing their passion for inquiry. Their expertise and enthusiasm can motivate aspiring researchers to pursue advanced studies and engage in innovative projects that address pressing challenges in paramedicine. By mentoring and providing guidance, established researchers can cultivate a supportive environment that fosters curiosity, critical thinking, and collaboration, ultimately ensuring a strong and progressive future for paramedic research.

> *"To those considering a career in research, I advise staying resilient, staying curious, and seeking out collaborations with peers and mentors who can inspire and support your growth. Every step forward not only enhances personal development but also advances knowledge and contributes to positive change in the field."*
>
> Case Study 5

Chapter Summary

Becoming a competent researcher is a journey that involves continuous learning and development. Whilst there is a need for formal education regarding research design and methodology, there are informal opportunities for aspiring competent paramedic researchers to engage in their own development, as well as contribute to that of the wider professional community. As well as designing and conducting their own research, competent researchers will also undertake project leadership—part of which supports the development of aspiring paramedic researchers.

Case Study 5

Name: Alanowd Alghaith

Job title: PhD Student | Teaching Assistant

Affiliation(s): University of Leicester, Social science APPlied Healthcare and Improvement REsearch (SAPPHIRE) Group, Department of Population Health Sciences, College of Life Sciences | King Saud bin Abdulaziz University for Health Sciences, Department of Emergency Medical Services, College of Applied Medical Science | King Abdullah International Medical Research Center, Riyadh, Saudi Arabia

Short biography of your career and key motivators for pursuing a research career.

I stared my career as a paramedic in 2020 after completing my bachelor's degree in emergency medical services (EMS). During my internship, I found myself constantly pondering how I could make a difference in the field of paramedicine. Especially that, during my shifts, I frequently encountered critically ill patients, which sparked my interest in resuscitation and critical care. It was a year of deep reflection, where I debated whether to delve deeper into clinical practice or explore the academic side to drive change through research.

The turning point came when an opportunity emerged to become a teaching assistant in EMS, a job that will provide me with the opportunity to purse my higher education. It was a tough decision to step away from hands-on patient care, but I realised academia offered a unique platform to improve pre-hospital care through evidence-based approaches.

After that, my passion for critical care drove me to specialise in this subject for my master's studies. Currently, I am doing my PhD research, which focuses on improving early identification of critically ill children. My journey is guided by a strong desire to make a lasting, positive impact on paramedicine and patient care overall.

A specific challenge you have faced pursuing and undertaking this stage of your career.
One of the main challenges I faced when I first started my academia was reading and critiquing research papers effectively. Initially, I struggled to distinguish between high-quality and poor-quality studies. To develop this critical skill, I undertook several methodology courses and read research methods books to better understand research design and analysis. Additionally, I looked at high-quality studies that were highlights in the field and looked how experts critiqued them. I then realised that gaining this skill required both a solid foundation in research knowledge and extensive reading in the field. This combination of education and practice significantly improved my ability to evaluate research critically.

Benefits/rewards of pursuing a career in research.
One of the most rewarding moments in my research career happened when I worked on a major project focused on launching the first Saudi Out of Hospital Cardiac Arrest Registry. Initially, many struggles were faced including protocol development, ethical considerations, and data collection across the country. However, when we finally presented our initial findings, it was incredibly fulfilling. I felt a deep sense of accomplishment knowing that

(continued)

(continued)

our work could serve as a cornerstone for future studies aimed at improving outcomes for these patients. Being part of developing a national registry felt like a significant contribution to the field, reinforcing my belief in the transformative power of research in healthcare.

Future plans and top tips/advice to others considering a career in research.
Currently, my primary focus is successfully completing my PhD program. Beyond that, I am committed to leading initiatives that develop and implement guidelines, protocols, and innovative approaches to enhance EMS. My ultimate goal is to influence the direction of prehospital care through impactful research.

To those considering a career in research, I advise staying resilient, staying curious, and seeking out collaborations with peers and mentors who can inspire and support your growth. Every step forward not only enhances personal development but also advances knowledge and contributes to positive change in the field.

Case Study 6

Name: Ryan Matthews

Job title: Lecturer and PhD Candidate

Affiliation(s): Cape Peninsula University of Technology and University of Cape Town

Short biography of your career.
I began giving earnest consideration to a career in research just after I had completed a master's degree and

had registered for a postgraduate teaching qualification. I had also just begun teaching at a university and while developing my class content I became frustrated by how underserved paramedicine is in terms of disciplinary knowledge. The lack of contextually relevant disciplinary knowledge made solving the clinical and educational problems I was encountering difficult. I applied my newly acquired research skills to the body of literature and produced little. When colleagues and other experts let me know that they too were struggling to find the answers they needed I realised the need for research.

And then, of course, there was the satisfaction that comes with discovery. A senior colleague and I were conducting research to inform on an educational problem our department was experiencing. Watching the data come in and take shape was thrilling. This experience and the obvious need for research set me on this path.

Key motivators for pursuing a research career.
Pursuing a research career was a process of realisation for me. There was no 'aha' moment where I decided this is what I wanted to do. It was a voyage of discovery and exploration, much like the research itself.

A specific challenge you have faced pursuing and undertaking this stage of your career.
Paramedicine is still forming a research culture. We have relatively few experienced researchers and disciplinary professors, especially in South Africa. This means research leadership and mentorship is sometimes difficult to find. As an early career researcher, undertaking projects on my own, or needing to supervise other

(continued)

(continued)

students can be intimidating and bewildering. Mentorship is crucial. Finding a mentor with whom I could hold honest, and sometimes humbling discussions, and with whom I could talk through problems was indispensable. Sometimes an alternate view from someone who understands how you make meaning of things is what is needed. Mentorship was the key for me.

Benefits/rewards of pursuing a career in research.
Research can be boring, and tedious, and monotonous, and difficult. While in the thick of it, it is easy to lose sight of the end goal and one sometimes wonders if it is worth it. I had reached that point when one day I found myself sitting in a presentation by a colleague. He was describing a similar educational problem to one I had researched and published on the year before, as a co-author. When he began discussing his proposed solutions, he cited our work as contributary. The worth and reward for research was made clear.

Future plans and top tips/advice to others considering a career in research.
My goal for my career is to focus my work into a research niche and to develop specific areas of the discipline.

The single lesson which has helped me on this journey is to adopt an explorer mindset. Initially I expected my projects to be clear cut, targeted, and to conform to an exquisitely detailed plan. Research is about problem solving, not 'answer finding'. An answer to a question might be the end product, but that answer is not just lying around waiting for you. Discovering, or constructing it, takes creative thinking, responsiveness, and adaptability as well as tenacity. Researchers need to become comfortable in the unknown and not be intimidated by uncertainty. If it were not like that, it would not be research.

Case Study 7

Name: Thomas Hofmann

Job title: Paramedic | Lecturer

Affiliation(s): HSD Hochschule Doepfer GmbH, Potsdam | German Society of Paramedic Science, Aachen | Universität Witten/Herdecke, Witten

Short biography of your career.
After paramedic training in 2002, I started studying business administration in 2006. Then and now it is not possible to study paramedicine with institutions of higher education in Germany. After finishing my bachelor's degree, I worked as a manager in different German ambulance services. However, I was still more interested in frontline roles. To gain more experience, I worked as frontline paramedic in Ghana, Denmark, and Germany while I pursued my master's in management. During that time, a small group and I found the German Society of Paramedic Science (DGRe) which wants to integrate science more and more into German paramedicine and to establish study programmes in paramedicine with German universities and universities of applied science. Thereafter, I started working towards my PhD in health service research. Currently I'm working on establishing a paramedicine top-up bachelor programme at a university of applied sciences.

Key motivators for pursuing a research career.
What German paramedics know and do is mainly based on physicians' perspectives and research. As a part of the

(continued)

(continued)

professionalisation, it is important to establish an own knowledge body for German paramedics.

A specific challenge you have faced pursuing and undertaking this stage of your career.

At the very beginning of research in paramedicine in Germany, there was a lot of scepticism from colleagues and physicians. It is still necessary to convince important stakeholder about the necessity of paramedic driven research. As the German ambulance system is organised on a very small scale, the relevant institutions have to be contacted for every piece of research and data collection. In some cases, the medical directors have to be painstakingly persuaded to make the data available.

Benefits/rewards of pursuing a career in research.

As a researcher, it might be one of the best experiences when you see that your research makes a difference. There were some occasions, where my work or the work of DGRe colleagues were cited in documents of the German Federal Ministry of Health or in a conference at the parliament—the Bundestag. To see, that political decisions with far-reaching consequences are based on the own work is very rewarding.

Future plans and top tips/advice to others considering a career in rwwesearch.

Until now, it is still not possible to study paramedicine in German. So, whoever considers a research career need to find a related academic area where research in paramedicine can be carried out. Furthermore, it is important that almost all research work—even bachelor or master theses—get published. Get in contact with fellow researches, visit conferences, build strong groups, and support each other. Paramedic science is at an important threshold in Germany, and we need collaboration to institutionalise it in Germany's universities and colleges.

Case Study 8

Name: Cheryl Cameron

Job title: Director of Operations | PhD Candidate | Senior Fellow

Affiliation(s): Department of Paramedicine, Monash University | Canadian Virtual Hospice | McNally Project for Paramedicine Research

Short biography of your career.
My journey started with a key turning point, although I didn't know it at the time. While considering quitting university to become a paramedic (paramedicine is not an undergraduate degree in Canada . . . yet), my dad crossed paths with a paramedic who suggested I finish my degree first. They could see the need for paramedicine to professionalise, and that to build a career leading that change, I needed more tools in my toolbox. Heeding this advice (thanks Vance!) laid the groundwork for my career path to date. I have served in various clinical and operational roles within urban and rural paramedic services, developed curriculum, and taught hundreds of paramedic students. I have led significant changes to practice, such as bringing palliative care approaches into paramedicine. I have held leadership positions in paramedic services, post-secondary institutions, and government, gaining experience in policy and governance. I currently serve as a senior leader in a national not-for-profit organisation, where we build digital resources and tools, co-designed with people with lived experience. I am passionate about optimising paramedicine's contribution to local communities and the larger healthcare system while mentoring and supporting others.

(continued)

(continued)

Key motivators for pursuing a research career.
I have always been a lifelong learner. Building capacity in research via a PhD seemed like a natural next step, so when an opportunity came up, I jumped at it. As a mentor and educator at heart, one of my key motivations is to build expertise in this space, so I can continue to support others.

A specific challenge you have faced pursuing and undertaking this stage of your career.
It is not about the academic work. If you have picked up this handbook, you can do it. You can learn new ways of thinking, develop new skills to approach problems, and synthesise what you have discovered. The greatest challenge is figuring out how to integrate the work into your overall life. Pursuing a PhD part time, working full time, raising a tiny human, staying physically and mentally healthy, and maintaining capacity to be a compassionate and supportive spouse, parent, colleague, and friend is the biggest challenge. Reflecting on what is important to you, who you are, what your goals are, and learning how to prioritise your needs is the challenging work. It is more about navigating the waters and adjusting as you go versus overcoming the challenge.

Benefits/rewards of pursuing a career in research.
The rewards are in the relationships. I have found inspiration to keep challenging myself (and to keep going) in the research community in paramedicine. I am forced to stretch and grow, and I know I can contribute and have an impact. I have found new friends, colleagues, and

collaborators, and have already had additional 'doors opened' because I said yes to pursuing the research arm of my career.

Future plans and top tips/advice to others considering a career in research. My current goal is completing my PhD, expanding my toolbox with new ways of thinking and solving problems.

One thing I've learned along my journey, is the importance of identifying your *why*. Identify your why. Why are you interested in this pathway? Is it for a specific career, is it to build an additional skill set, is it to influence or make change? Think about your why and revisit it often, as when things get hairy, it is the *why* that pulls you through and helps you to identify what you need to succeed.

Reach out, find your community, and build your circle of support, academically, professionally, and personally. You need a network of cheerleaders and supporters to help carry the load. It does take a village, so start building and broadening your personal and professional circle of support.

References

1. Gonzalez, E. and Forister, J. (2020). Conducting qualitative research. In: *Introduction to Research and Medical Literature*, 5e (ed. J. Forister and D. Blessing), 111–124. Information Age Publishing, Inc.
2. Paramedic Association of Canada (2024). PAC career framework for paramedics. https://doi.org/10.17605/OSF.IO/WDH9M (accessed 16 July 2024).

3. College of Paramedics (2024). *Paramedic Career Framework 2022 5th Edition Revised* https://collegeofparamedics.co.uk/COP/ProfessionalDevelopment/post_reg_career_frame work.aspx (accessed 19 December 2023).
4. NHS England and the National Institute for Health Research (2019). *12 actions to support and apply research in the NHS* [online] https://www.england.nhs.uk/wp-content/uploads/2018/05/12-actions-to-support-and-apply-research-i n-the-nhs.pdf

Further Reading

Greenhalgh, T.a.D.,.P. (2024). *How to Read a Paper: The Basics of Evidence-Based Medicine and Healthcare*, 7e. Wiley.
Punch, K. (2016). *Developing Effective Research Proposals*, 3e. Sage.

Chapter 6
Proficient Researcher

Walter Tavares
University of Toronto, Department of Health and Society, Toronto, Ontario, Canada

Chapter Objectives

1. Introduce the proficient researcher role and describe the transition from competent researcher.
2. Describe the key responsibilities, attributes, and support needs of a proficient researcher.

Research-focused Careers for Paramedics, First Edition.
Edited by Gregory A. Whitley and Scott Munro.

3. Define and contextualise proficiency in academic research, specifically within the domain of paramedicine, by integrating insights from multiple theoretical frameworks.

This chapter explores the concept of proficiency in the context of a research career. Drawing on multiple theoretical frameworks, it provides a comprehensive analysis of what constitutes proficiency. The chapter highlights the transition from competence to proficiency, which is marked by increased autonomy, leadership, reflective practice, and interdisciplinary collaboration. Key themes for proficient researchers, such as adaptability, problem-solving, mentorship, and practical application are explored in depth, providing a road map for aspiring researchers. The chapter aims to deepen the understanding of proficiency, emphasising its critical role in shaping research careers and contributing to increased research capacity and the advancement of paramedicine.

Proficiency, as a concept, refers to a high level of competence or expertise in a given skill or domain. It encompasses not only the acquisition of foundational knowledge but also the ability to apply that knowledge in a manner that is both efficient and effective. Proficiency implies mastery beyond basic or intermediate capabilities, where the individual can perform tasks autonomously, solve complex problems, and adapt to new situations within their field of expertise. This level of expertise often results from sustained practice, formal training, and reflective experience, wherein skills are refined and honed to meet high professional or academic standards.

In many fields, proficiency is recognised as the stage at which individuals can apply their knowledge with a degree of fluency and precision. They not only understand the theoretical frameworks underlying their work but can also navigate the practical challenges that arise in real-world applications. Furthermore, proficient individuals typically possess strong problem-solving abilities, enabling them to approach new or unforeseen circumstances with confidence and creativity. This adaptability is often what distinguishes proficiency from competency, as proficient individuals demonstrate an ability to innovate and refine their approaches in light of new challenges or contexts.

In research, proficiency represents a critical transition from being a participant or contributor to becoming a leader and innovator within a chosen field. Just as language proficiency enables a speaker to use nuanced expressions and adapt to varying communicative contexts, research proficiency allows a researcher to design and conduct studies autonomously, tackle complex research questions, and contribute original knowledge to their discipline. This stage is marked by an ability to manage research projects from inception to publication, including securing funding, overseeing research teams, and ensuring that findings have practical implications.

At the proficient level, researchers not only follow established methodologies but also critique and refine these approaches, introducing new techniques where necessary. Like the fluent speaker who adapts language use to context, the proficient researcher is adaptable, able to adjust their methods and approaches in response to the evolving needs of their study. Furthermore, proficient researchers possess the intellectual and managerial skills required to guide teams, navigate ethical complexities, and communicate findings effectively to both academic and non-academic audiences.

Thus, proficiency in research, like proficiency in language or any other skill, is not merely about performing tasks correctly but about mastering the art of applying knowledge creatively and confidently, pushing the boundaries of what is known, and contributing to the growth and development of the field.

Introduction to the Proficient Researcher Role

The proficient researcher in paramedicine represents a pivotal stage in a paramedic's research career. This phase is characterised by a significant shift from merely contributing to research efforts to taking a leading role in the entire research process [1]. No longer are proficient researchers focused solely on participation or research delivery; they are now responsible for the more advanced aspects of research leadership, study design, securing project funding, and managing research teams [2] (see **Figure 6.1**). This

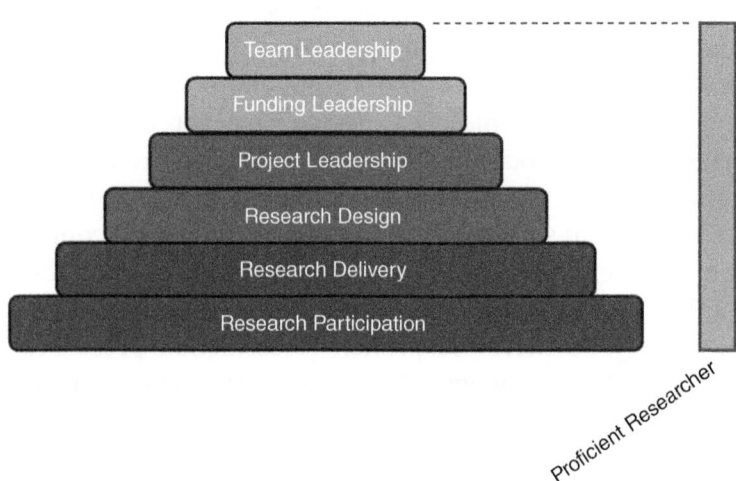

Figure 6.1 Proficient Researcher

evolution aligns loosely with postdoctoral achievements in the academic world, where researchers demonstrate independence and authority in their field [3].

At this level, proficient researchers are expected to lead projects that shape the future of paramedicine research. Their work not only contributes to the body of knowledge but also frequently influences policy and best practices at national and international levels [4]. By bridging the gap between the clinical practice of paramedicine and academic research, proficient researchers ensure that innovations derived from their studies are translated into actionable improvements in patient outcomes. This integration of research into practice is essential for evidence-based care, which directly impacts the quality of services provided by paramedics worldwide [4].

In addition to their clinical expertise, proficient researchers are equipped with the advanced technical skills necessary for every stage of research delivery. These skills extend beyond data collection and analysis to include securing competitive funding, managing diverse and interdisciplinary research teams, and overseeing complex, large-scale projects [5]. The ability to secure external funding is a particularly crucial skill at this level, as proficient researchers often lead multi-year studies that require significant financial resources [2].

Greater responsibility in decision-making also defines this stage. Proficient researchers are tasked with conceptualising research questions that address pressing clinical challenges in paramedicine. Their work begins with identifying gaps in current knowledge and extends to disseminating findings to the broader healthcare community, ensuring that their research has both practical and academic impact. This expanded scope of responsibility means that proficient researchers must not only have a thorough understanding of research methodologies but must also develop leadership and project management skills that enable them to navigate the complexities of large-scale research initiatives.

Transitioning from Competent to Proficient Researcher

The transition from a competent to a proficient researcher marks a significant milestone in a paramedic's research career. While competent researchers might primarily engage in existing research projects, contributing to data collection, analysis, and sometimes limited design elements, proficient researchers embrace a more autonomous and strategic role. This stage is characterised by a shift from working under the supervision of senior researchers to taking the lead in developing independent research projects. The proficient researcher begins to define the research questions, design methodologies, and take ownership of the research agenda and program.

A critical aspect of this transition is the development of independent research ideas. Proficient researchers identify gaps in the current body of knowledge and conceptualise studies that address those gaps. This requires a deep understanding of the field, as well as the ability to critically assess existing literature and anticipate the future needs. The move toward independence also demands a refined skill set in securing research funding. Proficient researchers lead the process, drafting proposals, applying for competitive grants, and ensuring that the financial aspects of their projects are robust and sustainable.

While novice researchers typically participate in existing projects and contribute to research delivery, and competent researchers typically lead on small- to medium-scale projects, proficient researchers tend to take on significant project and team leadership roles. The transition often involves moving from executing research under supervision to developing independent research ideas and securing funding to bring them to fruition. Proficient researchers not only design and manage their projects but also oversee research teams, often composed of more junior researchers, research paramedics, and interdisciplinary collaborators. This requires strong project management skills, including the ability to coordinate tasks, manage timelines, and ensure that all team members are working towards the same goals. Additionally, proficient researchers must be adept at navigating the ethical and regulatory frameworks that govern clinical research, ensuring that their studies meet the highest standards of safety and rigor.

This stage also involves an increased focus on dissemination. Proficient researchers are responsible not only for conducting research but also for ensuring that the findings are shared with the broader scientific and clinical community. This often means presenting at conferences, publishing in peer-reviewed journals, and engaging with stakeholders, including policymakers, to translate research into practice. The ability to effectively communicate research findings is essential for influencing policy and clinical guidelines, making this a crucial responsibility of the proficient researcher.

This transition from competent to proficient researcher is captured here:

> *"I studied for a BSc, started a secondment working as a trial coordinator on a head injury research study and then successfully applied again for the NIHR MClinRes. The initial 12-month secondment was extended and after that I never really left research. During my MClinRes I met Professor Chris Price and we got talking about stroke care. This eventually led to the Stroke Association funding my PhD and post-doctoral fellowship and seven to eight years work focussed on prehospital stroke care which all led to my current position."*
>
> Case Study 9

Responsibilities of the Proficient Researcher

The responsibilities that accompany this role are multifaceted and demanding, yet they offer immense rewards—both in personal satisfaction and in the tangible improvements made to the profession. The following section explores the specific responsibilities that define the proficient researcher, using real-world examples to illustrate how paramedics at this level lead and innovate within their field. In addition to research participation and research delivery (discussed in **Chapter 4**), research design and leadership (discussed in **Chapter 5**), at this stage, paramedics are also expected to have funding leadership and team leadership skills. Proficient researchers have an in-depth understanding of research methodologies and are capable of developing complex study protocols. They also navigate the administrative and ethical requirements of research, ensuring that projects adhere to regulatory standards.

As one paramedic researcher explains, this stage involves a balance between clinical responsibilities and leadership in research initiatives. Despite the challenges of balancing clinical shifts with research, proficient researchers thrive by setting clear boundaries and maintaining a structured routine:

"The flexibility of research is a double-edged sword. As a clinician dedicated to giving 100%, it was challenging to set boundaries regarding work hours and task loads, especially during my PhD. This period coincided with the height of the pandemic, where I juggled additional clinical shifts, home-schooling two children, and waking up at 5 a.m. to analyse qualitative data. Balancing these demands required a newfound discipline and resilience. Overcoming this challenge involved developing a structured routine, prioritizing tasks effectively, and seeking support from mentors and colleagues. This experience taught me the importance of time management and self-care in maintaining both personal and professional well-being."

Case Study 11

Funding Leadership

A major part of the proficient researcher's role is securing external funding for projects. This requires skills in writing grant applications, presenting research ideas to potential sponsors, and justifying the clinical relevance of the proposed study. Another paramedic researcher, for example, faced significant challenges in obtaining funding as paramedicine is still misunderstood and undervalued within the wider healthcare system. However, she overcame these obstacles by working with established researchers and applying for smaller grants before moving on to larger-scale projects:

> *"Paramedicine is very mis-understood, undervalued and overlooked within the greater healthcare system. This has made obtaining research funding even more challenging than it already is, and I was competing against expert researchers from more established fields with many more years of experience. This is where most research careers end. To overcome this, I worked on research teams for more established researchers. I wasn't always doing research I was passionate about, but I was developing my skills, and being listed on grants and publications. I also applied for smaller grants to pursue my research interests and between these two strategies, I have built my track record. This has led to success in larger funding applications."*
>
> Case Study 10

Team Leadership

Proficient researchers often lead interdisciplinary teams, coordinating efforts across various healthcare professionals, researchers, and institutions. Effective team management is crucial for the successful delivery of research, from recruiting participants to managing data collection and analysis. In many cases, proficient researchers work closely with paramedic teams, providing training and support to ensure the successful integration of research protocols into day-to-day clinical practice. Some paramedic researchers plan to develop bespoke research units to facilitate multidisciplinary team working:

> *"I hope to one day setup a prehospital research unit where researchers from diverse professional and personal backgrounds can come together to work on solutions for challenges faced by low- to middle-income countries."*
> Case Study 12

Frameworks for Proficiency in Research

In this section, I use the work of Timothy C. Guetterman to conceptually explore proficiency in research [6]. Dr. Guetterman is a researcher and academic known for his contributions to the field of mixed methods research, a methodological approach that integrates both qualitative and quantitative data. He has authored and co-authored numerous publications that focus on research methodologies, particularly within health sciences and education. My aim is not to position mixed methods research (or any other methodology) as an indicator of proficiency. Rather, his work on assessing and developing proficiency in mixed methods research, which was the subject of his 2015 doctoral dissertation, provides a useful framework by which to explore proficiency. Guetterman developed a framework to assess mixed methods research proficiency, which has been influential in advancing how researchers approach proficiency, in this case for mixed methods research, ensuring that they can more effectively engage in research to answer complex research questions [6].

Guetterman's framework [6] provides valuable insights into the broader process of becoming a proficient researcher, particularly in fields like paramedicine where both qualitative and quantitative data play crucial roles. Proficiency in this type of research, according to Guetterman, hinges on several key factors: professional experience, knowledge, skills, and personal characteristics. These elements align closely with the path to proficiency in paramedic research, where researchers must not only understand multiple methodologies but also apply them well. Guetterman highlights the importance of professional experience in building proficiency, emphasising that real-world application is central to mastering it. This aligns with the broader notion that proficient researchers must engage actively in research projects, learning through practice rather than theory alone. As with paramedic research, hands-on experience in mixed methods is invaluable for understanding how to design studies that answer complex questions, manage large datasets, and integrate diverse findings into coherent conclusions.

Moreover, knowledge and skills are essential to achieving proficiency [6]. Guetterman's framework emphasises that researchers must have a deep understanding of both qualitative and quantitative research methodologies, as well as the ability to combine these approaches effectively. This parallels the requirements in paramedic research, where proficiency involves mastering not only clinical and medical knowledge but also advanced research methodologies and data analysis techniques. Researchers at this level are expected to lead the design of studies, navigate ethical and logistical challenges, and ensure rigorous execution of research protocols.

Perhaps one of the most salient aspects of Guetterman's framework is the focus on personal characteristics—such as persistence, adaptability, and critical thinking—as vital to achieving proficiency [6]. These traits enable researchers to navigate the inevitable challenges that arise during complex research projects, including managing time, securing funding, and balancing research with other professional duties. In paramedic research, these personal qualities are equally important, as proficient researchers often work in fast-paced, high-pressure environments where they must be both flexible and methodical.

Finally, Guetterman's framework introduces the concept of self-assessment as a tool for developing proficiency [6]. By reflecting on their strengths and areas for growth, researchers can identify where additional training or experience is needed, whether in mastering specific methodologies or improving their leadership and project management skills. In paramedic research, this type of self-assessment can be particularly valuable, allowing researchers to track their progress as they take on increasingly complex studies and leadership roles.

In summary, Guetterman's framework provides a robust model for understanding and developing research proficiency, particularly in interdisciplinary fields like mixed methods research. The integration of knowledge, experience, and personal attributes creates a pathway for researchers to progress from novice to proficient, ultimately enabling them to lead projects that push the boundaries of what is known in their field.

Additional Frameworks for Understanding Proficiency in Research

Achieving proficiency as a researcher involves integrating knowledge, skills, and personal development. Several key frameworks provide insights into the nature of research proficiency and the journey from competence to expertise (See Table 6.1).

Table 6.1 Frameworks guiding insights related to proficiency in research

Framework	Proficiency in Research
The Dreyfus Model (1980), developed by Stuart and Hubert Dreyfus, outlines a five-stage progression: novice, advanced beginner, competent, proficient, and expert.	In the context of research, proficiency is characterised by the ability to navigate complex tasks independently, apply intuition, and think beyond procedural rules. Proficient researchers recognise patterns holistically and approach problems with adaptive and flexible strategies, moving beyond rule-based decisions. This model provides a valuable perspective on the shift from dependence on structured guidelines to a more fluid, experience-driven approach.
Ernest Boyer (1990) [7] proposed a framework to understand the diverse roles of researchers in academia. Boyer's Model categorises research proficiency into four types of scholarship: discovery, integration, application, and teaching.	Proficient researchers contribute significantly in each of these areas: • *Discovery*: Conducting original research to expand the body of knowledge. • *Integration*: Synthesising information across disciplines to generate new insights. • *Application*: Applying knowledge to solve practical, real-world problems. • *Teaching*: Sharing and disseminating research findings to educate others. Boyer's Model emphasises the importance of both generating new knowledge and sharing that knowledge effectively, which is crucial for proficient researchers seeking to impact practice and policy.

Table 6.1 (continued)

Framework	Proficiency in Research
Kolb's Experiential Learning Theory (1984) [8] outlines learning as a continuous cycle involving concrete experience, reflective observation, abstract conceptualisation, and active experimentation.	Proficient researchers engage deeply in each of these stages. They learn through hands-on research experiences, reflect on the outcomes, conceptualise improvements, and actively apply these lessons in subsequent projects. This iterative process is central to achieving research proficiency and refining skills over time.
Donald Schön (1983) [9] highlights the role of reflection in professional practice.	Proficient researchers are reflective practitioners who critically analyse their work throughout the research process. By reflecting in action (during research activities) and on action (after completing research), proficient researchers continually refine their methodologies and approaches. This reflective practice allows them to adapt effectively to new challenges and is key to evolving from competent to proficient levels.
Lev Vygotsky's Zone of Proximal Development (1978) [10] suggests that individuals develop proficiency through social interactions with more knowledgeable mentors.	In the context of research, mentoring relationships are instrumental in helping researchers advance their skills. Proficient researchers have often benefitted from guidance provided by mentors, which helps them tackle tasks just beyond their current abilities, pushing them towards greater independence and expertise.

(continued)

Table 6.1 (continued)

Framework	Proficiency in Research
The National Institute for Health Research (NIHR) Clinical Academic Career Framework [2] provides a structured pathway for healthcare professionals, including paramedics, to develop research careers. This framework outlines progression from novice to expert researcher, with proficiency being a crucial intermediate stage.	Proficient researchers are expected to take leadership roles, manage interdisciplinary research teams, and ensure that research findings are translated into clinical practice. This framework emphasises the integration of research and clinical skills, which is particularly relevant for paramedicine.
Kunihiko Hatano and Keiko Inagaki's (1986) [11] adaptive expertise suggests that unlike routine experts, who rely on mastered skills and habitual responses, adaptive experts are able to adjust their approaches, innovate, and solve novel problems effectively.	Adaptive expertise involves both efficiency—the ability to execute tasks quickly and accurately—and innovation—the capacity to think creatively and modify existing practices to address new challenges. Proficient researchers go beyond routine application of established procedures. They are flexible, question assumptions, and seek new methods to overcome research barriers.

Common Themes Across Frameworks

Despite their varied origins and applications, these frameworks share several common themes that help define research proficiency (see **Figure 6.2**):

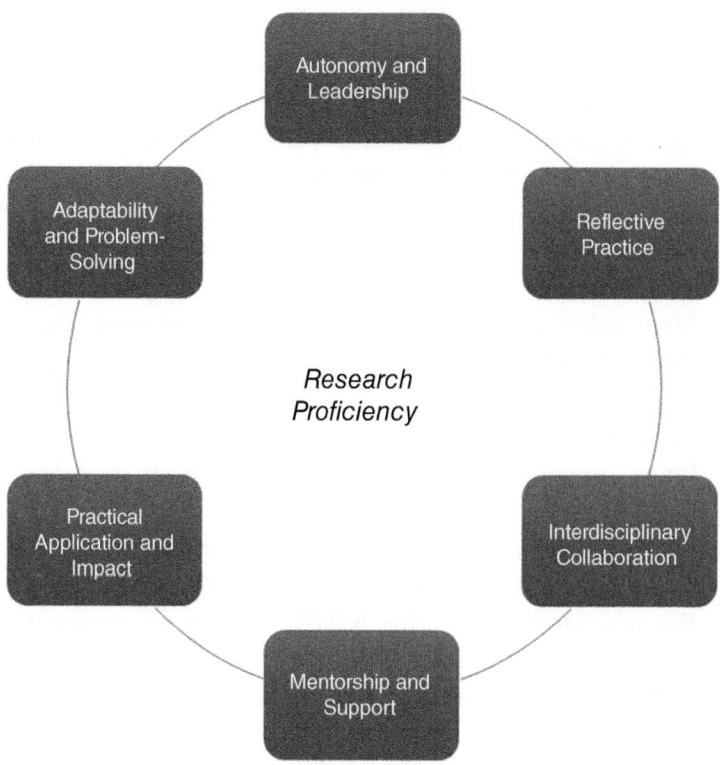

Figure 6.2 Themes of Research Proficiency

1. *Autonomy and Leadership*: Proficient researchers transition from dependency on guidance to leading their own research projects. They demonstrate autonomy in designing, conducting, and disseminating research, often taking on leadership roles that involve mentoring others and managing teams.
2. *Reflective Practice*: Reflection is crucial in developing proficiency. Researchers engage in continuous reflection, both during and after their research activities, to identify areas for improvement and adapt their approaches.

Schön's and Kolb's frameworks particularly emphasise the importance of reflection for learning and growth.

3. *Interdisciplinary Collaboration*: Proficiency often requires working across disciplines. Boyer's Model and the NIHR framework highlight the need for researchers to synthesise knowledge from various fields and collaborate with diverse experts to address complex research questions effectively.

4. *Mentorship and Support*: Mentorship is a recurring theme in developing proficiency, as highlighted by Vygotsky's ZPD (Zone of Proximal Development). Support from experienced mentors helps researchers navigate challenges, expand their skill set, and transition to more independent roles.

5. *Practical Application and Impact*: Proficient researchers strive to make their work applicable beyond academia. Boyer's Model and the NIHR framework stress the importance of translating research into practice, thereby bridging the gap between theory and clinical application to improve patient outcomes.

6. *Adaptability and Problem-Solving*: Proficient researchers are characterised by their adaptability and ability to solve problems creatively. The Dreyfus Model and Kolb's Experiential Learning Theory emphasise that proficiency involves responding to challenges with innovative and flexible solutions, which is critical in the dynamic environment of paramedic research.

Personal Attributes and Support Needs of Proficient Researchers

Next, we consider potential progression pathways of paramedic researchers towards proficiency, which often obligate blending personal attributes with necessary external support while also balancing between internal drive and institutional resources.

Proficient researchers in paramedic research share a range of personal qualities, skills, and experiences that drive their success. Central to their proficiency is a strong work ethic and deep dedication to their research. These individuals are not easily deterred by setbacks; instead, they demonstrate resilience and perseverance, continuously pushing forward in their pursuit of new knowledge. What truly sets them apart is their intrinsic motivation—rather than being driven solely by external incentives such as recognition or funding, they find personal satisfaction and fulfilment in the research process itself. For proficient researchers, the act of inquiry, the search for answers, and the potential to improve patient care are rewards in their own right.

Another critical factor in attaining research proficiency is the rigorous training in research methodology and academic writing that many researchers gain through structured programs, such as doctoral studies. This training equips them with the skills necessary to design robust research studies, conduct comprehensive analyses, and effectively disseminate their findings. The ability to communicate research outcomes, both in writing and presentations, is vital for contributing to the academic community and influencing clinical practice.

Time management is another key to proficiency. Proficient researchers must be adept at balancing the demands of research with other responsibilities, such as clinical practice, teaching, or administrative duties. They prioritise their research by allocating dedicated time to it, often developing structured work habits—such as regular writing and data analysis schedules—that ensure steady progress. Proficiency in research is not achieved overnight, and effective time management allows these researchers to maintain consistent output over the long term.

Access to resources and support from colleagues also plays an instrumental role in the development of research proficiency. Mentorship from experienced researchers can provide guidance, encouragement, and critical feedback, helping researchers refine their ideas and methodologies. Collaborative opportunities, both within their institutions and internationally, expose them to new perspectives and foster a culture of shared knowledge and innovation. These networks are invaluable for sparking new ideas, finding research partners, and gaining constructive insights.

The institutional environment further influences research proficiency. Proficient researchers often thrive in institutions that prioritise research and provide necessary resources such as funding, research assistants, and technical support. Importantly, institutions that protect time for research by limiting teaching and administrative duties enable researchers to fully focus on their projects, which is crucial for driving significant research progress. Institutions that foster a research culture—one that values inquiry, provides the infrastructure for experimentation, and rewards academic output—create fertile ground for researchers to excel.

Additionally, proficient researchers are strategic about their publication choices. They understand that publishing in high-quality, peer-reviewed journals enhances the visibility and impact of their work. By targeting reputable outlets aligned with their research area, they ensure that their findings reach relevant audiences and contribute to ongoing academic discussions. This strategic approach to publication is not only essential for advancing their careers but also for influencing clinical guidelines and policies in paramedicine.

Finally, staying connected to real-world issues and current events is critical. Proficient researchers keep a close watch on emerging challenges within their field and adapt their research to address pressing concerns. By aligning their work with significant issues in paramedicine, they ensure that their research is both academically relevant and practically useful, ultimately contributing to improvements in patient outcomes and service delivery.

While external support from institutions and colleagues is crucial, many of the most influential factors lie within the researchers themselves. Personal motivation, dedication, and the ability to manage time effectively are indispensable qualities that enable paramedics to become proficient researchers and make lasting contributions to the field.

Chapter Summary

The journey to becoming a proficient researcher is marked by an intricate blend of skills, experiences, and personal attributes. Across various frameworks, proficiency is consistently associated with the transition from structured learning and participation in projects to leading research endeavours, making independent decisions, and contributing new insights to the field. It involves moving beyond technical expertise to include leadership, reflective practice, and adaptability—qualities that enable researchers to navigate the uncertainties of complex inquiries.

Proficient researchers are characterised by their ability to identify meaningful research questions, design studies that bridge theoretical gaps, and apply their findings in real-world contexts. They not only excel in methodological rigor but also demonstrate the resilience and intrinsic motivation necessary to sustain long-term research careers. Institutional support, mentorship, and access to resources play crucial roles, but ultimately, it is the researchers' own drive and dedication that propel them to proficiency.

Proficiency also involves a heightened capacity for critical thinking and problem-solving. Proficient researchers are able to anticipate potential challenges in their studies, develop creative solutions, and adapt their methodologies as needed. This flexibility is essential, especially in fields where research contexts are dynamic and ever-changing. Furthermore, proficient researchers are not just contributors; they are leaders who inspire and mentor others, fostering a culture of inquiry and collaboration within their teams and broader communities.

In paramedic research, as in other fields, proficiency has a significant impact on both practice and policy. It enhances the capacity for evidence-based decision-making, informs clinical protocols, and ultimately leads to better patient outcomes. Proficient researchers translate complex data into actionable insights that can directly influence healthcare delivery. By doing so, they help bridge the gap between theory and practice, ensuring that research findings are implemented in ways that improve patient care and system efficiency.

The journey to proficiency is not without its challenges. Researchers must navigate the complexities of securing funding, managing interdisciplinary teams, and maintaining the balance between clinical duties and research activities. However, these challenges also present opportunities for growth. Through perseverance and effective time management, proficient researchers develop the resilience needed to overcome obstacles and continue pushing the boundaries of their field.

By embracing the combination of personal motivation, practical experience, rigorous training, and collaborative engagement, proficient researchers are not just advancing their own careers; they are actively shaping the future of paramedicine and contributing to a culture of continual improvement in healthcare. Their work not only advances scientific understanding but also directly impacts the quality of care provided to patients, ensuring that healthcare systems evolve in response to emerging needs and challenges.

Case Studies

Case Study 9

Name: Graham McClelland

Job title: Vice Chancellors' Fellow | Honorary Research Fellow | Visiting Clinical Researcher | Visiting Professor

Affiliation(s): Northumbria University | North East Ambulance Service | Newcastle University | University of Hertfordshire

Short biography of your career.
I joined the ambulance service with no degree and no intention of going into research. A key turning point for me was seeing a MClinRes fellowship advertised which allowed you to study whilst working and getting paid

(continued)

(continued)

which was an amazing opportunity especially as I could see how my lack of a degree was becoming an issue. I applied for this scheme but was unsuccessful but the idea of getting involved in research never left.

I studied for a BSc, started a secondment working as a trial coordinator on a head injury research study and then successfully applied again for the National Institute for Health and Care Research (NIHR) MClinRes. The initial 12-month secondment was extended and after that I never really left research.

During my MClinRes, I met Professor Chris Price and we got talking about stroke care. This eventually led to the Stroke Association funding my PhD and postdoctoral fellowship and seven to eight years work focussed on pre-hospital stroke care which all led to my current position.

Key motivators for pursuing a research career.
I think my first post supporting a head injury pathways study (HITS-NS) really opened my eyes to the lack of evidence in pre-hospital care, the potential for evidence to influence care and the fact that other paramedics like me were interested in similar things and trying to do research as well.

A specific challenge you have faced pursuing and undertaking this stage of your career.
A huge challenge for me was the decision whether to leave the ambulance service to pursue research at a university. My ideal job had one foot in the ambulance service and one foot in a university; however, this was difficult to find/create. Towards the end of my postdoctoral

fellowship, I was thinking about what to do next and saw a university-based role that looked attractive and would allow me to keep developing as a researcher. Leaving the National Health Service (NHS) and the ambulance service after 20 years was a hard choice, but I felt there were limited development opportunities in the ambulance service, and it was the best move for me.

Benefits/rewards of pursuing a career in research.
One project I found very rewarding was the SATIATED2 project looking at the SALAD (Suction Assisted Laryngo-scopy Airway Decontamination) technique for managing a difficult airway which built on work by Richard Pilbery and co in YAS (Yorkshire Ambulance Service). Travelling around the North East training paramedics in the technique was really good fun all the while collecting data about their airway skills and the impact of SALAD. The real pay-off from this was when I started receiving emails from people saying they had used SALAD in practice and that it had helped their patients. It was really nice to be involved in something with such a direct impact on patient care.

Future plans and top tips/advice to others considering a career in research.
My top tip for any paramedic considering a career in research is go find the other people working in the field. There may not be lots of paramedics in any one service doing research, but there is a community of people out there doing research and finding them will open doors and provide opportunities for you to get involved in things. Nearly everyone I have met over the past 10+ years has been happy to talk about their research and willing to help when asked.

Case Study 10

Name: Kathryn Eastwood ASM

Job title: Associate Professor and Intensive Care Paramedic

Affiliation(s): Monash University

Short biography of your career.
I started my paramedic training in 2000 at Monash University. I concurrently finished a science degree in biochemistry and a Nursing degree that I'd started before being selected for the paramedic course. Because of my educational background, the day after I qualified as a paramedic, I was offered a position teaching the paramedic students anatomy, physiology, and pathophysiology. In 2005, I completed my intensive care paramedic (ICP) training and then completed a master's degree where I did my first research project. I was offered a lecturer position in 2009 whilst pregnant with my first child, and I continued to work part time as an ICP. In 2010, I started my PhD part time after having my second child (with a 16-month-old and 2-week-old!).

Seven years later, I completed my PhD. I was offered a position in the Department of Epidemiology and Preventive Medicine at Monash University where I continue to work today in addition to working as an ICP in Victoria, Australia.

Key motivators for pursuing a research career.
Even during my PhD candidature, I never really considered continuing in research. However, I was offered a Research Fellow position, so I decided to take the position

for a year then re-evaluate. Six years later, I'm still here and loving my work.

A specific challenge you have faced pursuing and undertaking this stage of your career.
Paramedicine is very misunderstood, undervalued, and overlooked within the greater healthcare system. This has made obtaining research funding even more challenging than it already is, and I was competing against expert researchers from more established fields with many more years of experience. This is where most research careers end.

To overcome this, I worked on research teams for more established researchers. I wasn't always doing research I was passionate about, but I was developing my skills and being listed on grants and publications. I also applied for smaller grants to pursue my research interests, and between these two strategies, I have built my track record. This has led to success in larger funding applications.

Benefits/rewards of pursuing a career in research.
It is very rewarding when I am invited into larger groups of multidisciplinary academics who I find intimidating, yet who genuinely value my role and the knowledge and experience I bring to our discussions. An example was being selected for the International Liaison Committee on Resuscitation (ILCOR), which is limited to around 150 global leading experts on resuscitation from all areas of medicine.

Other rewarding aspects include seeing my research making an impact on patients or the workforce and

(continued)

(continued)

assisting novice and competent researchers in their development.

Future plans and top tips/advice to others considering a career in research.

I feel being a researcher is a continuous process of learning and developing. Therefore, my goal is to continue to become a researcher that produces high-quality, impactful knowledge. My advice to others would be to get involved. Approach a research academic and ask to be included in a project. Research can be long and slow, so they need to be patient, but it is rewarding when your work is finally published. For those already in research, my advice is to keep striving to improve the quality of your research. And finally, if you start a PhD with two babies, seek psychological assistance urgently.

Case Study 11

Name: Caitlin Wilson

Job title: Senior Research Fellow (Paramedic)

Affiliation(s): Yorkshire Ambulance Service NHS Trust | University of Hertfordshire

Short biography of your career.

My career began in 2012 as a paramedic with North West Ambulance Service NHS Trust, following a two-year DipHE in Paramedic Practice, later topped up to a BSc. Even as a student, my ambition was to pursue a PhD, though I initially thought I was the only paramedic with a research interest. I quickly discovered otherwise while undertaking an NIHR-funded MSc in Clinical Research Methods in 2015/2016. My first conference at the 999 EMS Research Forum was a pivotal moment—I was amazed by the breadth of paramedic-related research. This inspired me to work as a research paramedic on the NIHR-funded PASTA (Paramedic Acute Stroke Treatment Assessment) trial before embarking on a PhD funded by an NIHR infrastructure studentship. I supplemented this by working one shift per week as an operational paramedic. Upon completing my PhD, I transitioned into a senior research fellow role, working across Yorkshire Ambulance Service NHS Trust and the University of Hertfordshire.

Key motivators for pursuing a research career.
I was always that curious student paramedic questioning 'why' we did things. I couldn't accept the answer: "That's just how we've always done it." Research allows me to delve deeper into the 'why' of paramedic practice and find ways to enhance patient care.

A specific challenge you have faced pursuing and undertaking this stage of your career.
The flexibility of research is a double-edged sword. As a clinician dedicated to giving 100%, it was challenging to set boundaries regarding work hours and task loads, especially during my PhD. This period coincided with the height of the pandemic, where I juggled additional clinical shifts, home-schooling two children, and waking up at 5 a.m. to analyse qualitative data. Balancing these demands required a new-found discipline and resilience. Overcoming this challenge involved developing a structured routine, prioritizing tasks

(continued)

(continued)

effectively, and seeking support from mentors and colleagues. This experience taught me the importance of time management and self-care in maintaining both personal and professional well-being.

Benefits/rewards of pursuing a career in research.
The rewards of research are profound. My top three moments include conducting my first qualitative interview, being invited to update the Joint Royal Colleges Ambulance Liaison Committee (JRCALC) guideline on hyperventilation syndrome following my MSc study, and discovering that paramedic students were critically appraising one of my publications as an assignment. Each of these moments reaffirmed the impact and value of my work. Additionally, seeing the practical applications of my research in clinical settings and knowing that my findings can directly improve patient care is incredibly fulfilling. Presenting at conferences and collaborating with other researchers also provides a sense of community and shared purpose, further enriching my career.

Future plans and top tips/advice to others considering a career in research.
Having achieved my long-time goal of obtaining a PhD, I now aim to solidify my career as a clinical–academic paramedic, balancing clinical shifts with ongoing research. My advice is to think creatively—if your dream job in paramedic research doesn't exist, take the initiative to create it. Network with like-minded professionals, seek out mentorship, and never stop questioning the status quo. Embrace challenges as opportunities for growth and remain passionate about the potential of your work to drive positive change. With dedication and perseverance, you can carve out a unique and impactful career path in paramedic research.

Case Study 12

Name: Willem Stassen

Job title: Associate Professor

Affiliation(s): Division of Emergency Medicine; Department of Family, Community and Emergency Care; University of Cape Town; South Africa

Short biography of your career.
I graduated as a degreed paramedic in 2010 from the University of Johannesburg. My first publication was on my graduate research. Back then, there were very few degreed paramedics in South Africa, and this meant that I covered multiple roles early on. This provided opportunities to see our emergency care system from multiple perspectives.

After a few months as a primary response paramedic, I joined a critical care retrieval service. My clinical experiences underscored the need for development and research in this field. I completed my master's at the University of Cape Town and moved to full-time helicopter emergency medical services. When that service closed, I moved to the dispatch centre, where another research interest developed. Here, I also lead a research unit which focused on solving relevant problems. In 2018, I completed my PhD at Karolinska Institute. While completing my master's and PhD, I started supervising student research. In 2018, I joined the University of Cape Town as the PhD programme convenor and emergency care researcher.

Key motivators for pursuing a research career.
Recognising the limitations of clinical work to effect systemic change motivated me to enter a research career. Clinical work impacts individuals, but to

(continued)

(continued)

impact the system, one has to find out more about the problems and think of ways to fix them. This is what researchers do.

A specific challenge you have faced pursuing and undertaking this stage of your career.
For my PhD, I naively planned to do one of the first prehospital randomised controlled trials in Africa. It didn't go very well, but I learnt a lot from it. We are still trying to successfully undertake one here in South Africa, but what I have come to learn was that research wheels can sometimes turn slowly when you are doing things that no one has tried before. It is therefore essential to sometimes first do some preliminary studies to understand the context better and to ensure that you do research for which the system is ready and can support.

Benefits/rewards of pursuing a career in research.
Pursuing a research career offers the privilege to connect with public and professional communities to address challenges that seem exceedingly complex. Due to this complexity, solutions often require a multifaceted approach, using various studies from multiple perspectives or methodological approaches. It is incredibly rewarding when you see multiple results come together to give you a fuller, more crystalised picture of what you are dealing with. This clarity can then be leveraged to devise practical solutions. These moments exemplify the true value and fulfilment that research pursuits bring.

Future plans and top tips/advice to others considering a career in research.

I hope to one day setup a pre-hospital research unit where researchers from diverse professional and personal backgrounds can come together to work on solutions for challenges faced by low- to middle-income countries.

Until then, I can offer the following tips for people considering a research career. Firstly, be familiar with multiple methodological approaches because solving complex problems requires different perspectives. Secondly, always collaborate, don't compete because we can do so much more when we put our minds and resources together. Lastly, find yourself a good sponsor that will actively advocate for your advancement and exposure to opportunities.

References

1. National Institute for Health Research (NIHR) (2015). *Building a Research Career: A Guide for Aspiring Clinical Academics and Their Managers.* National Institute for Health Research.
2. Creswell, J.W. (2013). *Research Design: Qualitative, Quantitative, and Mixed Methods Approaches.* Sage Publications.
3. Dreyfus, H.L. and Dreyfus, S.E. (1980). *A Five-Stage Model of the Mental Activities Involved in Directed Skill Acquisition.* Operations Research Center, University of California, Berkeley.
4. Kitson, A.L., Harvey, G., and McCormack, B. (1998). Enabling the implementation of evidence based practice: a conceptual framework. *Quality in Health Care 7* (3): 149–158.
5. Fraser, S.W. and Greenhalgh, T. (2001). Coping with complexity: educating for capability. *BMJ 323* (7316): 799–803.

6. Guetterman, T. C. (2015). Development of a self-assessment for research proficiency in mixed methods research: the mixed methods research proficiency scale. Doctoral dissertation, University of Nebraska-Lincoln.

7. Boyer, E.L. (1990). *Scholarship Reconsidered: Priorities of the Professoriate.* Princeton University Press, The Carnegie Foundation for the Advancement of Teaching.

8. Kolb, D.A. (1984). *Experiential Learning: Experience as the Source of Learning and Development.* Prentice-Hall.

9. Schön, D.A. (1983). *The Reflective Practitioner: How Professionals Think in Action.* Basic Books.

10. Vygotsky, L.S. (1978). *Mind in Society: The Development of Higher Psychological Processes.* Harvard University Press.

11. Hatano, G. and Inagaki, K. (1986). Two courses of expertise. In: *Child Development and Education in Japan* (ed. H. Stevenson, H. Azuma, and K. Hakuta), 262–272. W. H. Freeman.

Further Reading

While the suggested readings below do not speak to the development of research proficiency directly, and certainly not in paramedicine specifically, they each provide important insights that can be applied to this concept, theoretically and practically.

Schön, D.A. (1983). *The Reflective Practitioner: How Professionals Think in Action.* Basic Books.
[Schön's work on reflective practice is crucial for understanding how researchers at the proficient level should engage in continual self-evaluation to refine their methods.]

Boyer, E.L. (1990). *Scholarship Reconsidered: Priorities of the Professoriate.* Princeton University Press.
[Boyer's framework can offer a broad view of research proficiency, highlighting the importance of scholarship in discovery, integration, application, and teaching.]

Guetterman, T. C. (2015). Development of a self-assessment for research proficiency in mixed methods research: the mixed

methods research proficiency scale. Doctoral dissertation, University of Nebraska-Lincoln.
[A valuable resource on assessing proficiency in mixed methods research, relevant for understanding broader concepts of proficiency in interdisciplinary research.]

Kolb, D.A. (1984). *Experiential Learning: Experience as the Source of Learning and Development.* Prentice-Hall.
[Kolb's experiential learning theory provides a useful framework for understanding how researchers can develop proficiency through cycles of concrete experience, reflection, and experimentation.]

Dreyfus, H.L. and Dreyfus, S.E. (1980). *A Five-Stage Model of the Mental Activities Involved in Directed Skill Acquisition.* Berkeley: University of California.
[This model outlines the progression from novice to expert, offering insights into the stages of skill acquisition relevant to developing research proficiency.]

Chapter 7

Expert Researcher

Peter O'Meara[1] and Malcolm Boyle[2]

[1] Monash University, Department of Paramedicine, Melbourne, Victoria, Australia

[2] Griffith University, School of Medicine and Dentistry, Gold Coast, Queensland, Australia

Research-focused Careers for Paramedics, First Edition.
Edited by Gregory A. Whitley and Scott Munro.
© 2025 John Wiley & Sons Ltd. Published 2025 by John Wiley & Sons Ltd.

Chapter Objectives

1. Examine and reflect on the place of expert paramedicine researchers in those countries where paramedicine researchers have been enabled to lead departments.
2. Consider why it is important that expert paramedicine researchers and their research findings are able to influence policy and practice amongst paramedics and the organisations where paramedics are employed.
3. Reflect on the rewards and challenges of being or becoming an expert researcher in paramedicine. Because of their rarity and recent emergence, it is likely that there will be some misunderstandings or debate about the nature and characteristics of expert researchers in paramedicine. Through this chapter, we aim to minimise this amongst our readers.

> *"I feel like my life has been about climbing mountains. That is, I had a goal (e.g., do a master's degree) and climbed that mountain. When I got to the top there were many other mountains I had not seen before. Each one I climbed led me to a place where there were many new mountains."*
>
> Case Study 14

The case studies presented in this chapter recognise that paramedicine researchers undertake and experience their own individual journeys toward being recognised as expert researchers. Their stories illustrate how specific roles and expectations vary according to individual circumstances and the environments in which individuals operate. For instance, while many expert paramedicine researchers will have full-time university appointments, others will hold honorary appointments alongside their other roles within pre-hospital organisations or with other employers. Our case studies highlight the diversity of career paths, research interests, and motivations that have emerged amongst the current generation of expert paramedicine researchers. Something these expert paramedic researchers may have experienced was a lack of guidance or mentorship in their early years, something which has changed over time where today there are experienced paramedicine researchers to guide new and emerging researchers.

In all three case studies, our contributors from three different countries commenced their paramedicine careers as trainee paramedics, emergency medical technicians (EMTs) or ambulance officers. Their pathways varied through unique twists and turns as result of design, fate or serendipity. They all demonstrated vision, curiosity, and perseverance as they obtained their doctoral qualifications and worked their way into positions where they could undertake and ultimately lead paramedicine-related research. In time, they were all recognised by their peers as expert researchers.

What Is an Expert Paramedic Researcher?

One common question posed is, what do we mean by the term expert researcher? Philosophers have been attempting to define what an expert is since the days of Plato [1]. Some argue that it is the nature of the role being undertaken that determines the answer to this query. The key factor in the eyes of Croce is that a real cognitive expert contributes to the epistemic progress of their discipline [2]. That is, the creation of new knowledge and insight of relevance to the profession across the domains of practice. This is an important distinction to make between those whose main role is that of sharing knowledge with laypersons and presumably students. Without going down that rabbit hole, we will concentrate on a working definition of expert researchers in paramedicine as seen by themselves and others in the field.

Paramedicine is now mature enough to have expert researchers associated with universities, research institutes, and health organisations, as well as a growing cohort of 'retired' paramedicine researchers who are recognised as sages to some degree. At this juncture, it is worth reiterating that research is both a pillar of professional practice and an integral component of professionalism alongside, education, self-regulation, building a professional knowledge base, and guiding management and clinical practice [3]. It is hard to argue that paramedicine is a profession in the absence of our own body of knowledge.

The main load for the creation of this body of knowledge falls to the research community alongside the organisations and practicing paramedics who implement and evaluate changes in policy and clinical practice. Expert researchers have a key role in research design and analysis of findings, as well as the important task of disseminating the outcomes. Expert researchers are also charged with the responsibility of mentoring new and emerging researchers to increase the pool of paramedicine researchers and encouraging creativity and innovation.

Considering the diversity of individual experiences, the description of a typical expert researcher in paramedicine is likely to remain elusive. However, there are arguably some shared experiences amongst those who are seen as expert researchers in our discipline. Amongst these is their

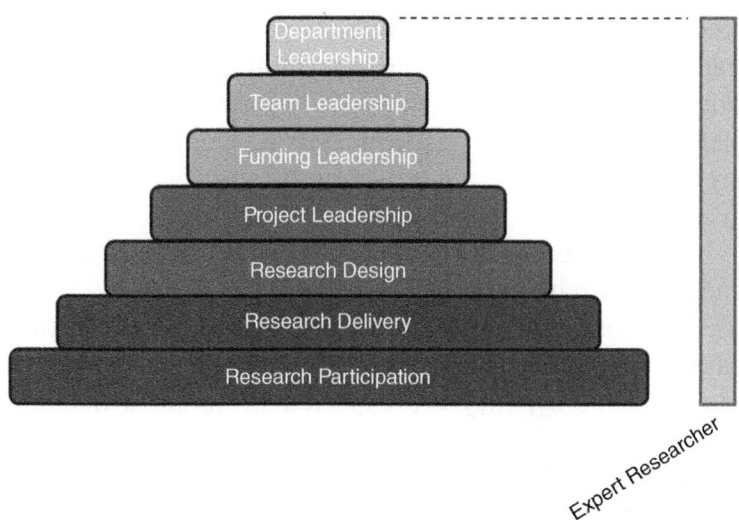

Figure 7.1 Expert Researcher

experience of progressing from a novice researcher to an expert (see **Figure 7.1**).

For the new academic researcher, entry into academia and the research world has typically come after a successful career across other professional domains of practice in ambulance services or other kindred organisations that employ paramedics [4]. This characteristic is shared with many others in the health professions, education, and business amongst others. Far fewer academics lack professional and life experience than the popular media would have us believe. As a result of this transition from industry to academia, many paramedics face challenges to their professional identity and status [4, 5]. They might be moving from a situation where they are at the 'top of their profession' to a situation where they feel that they are novices in an environment where conventions, policies, and cultural traditions are very different to the typical ambulance service. They may experience the 'imposter syndrome': they might feel inadequate in the academic domain, compared to their previous status as an experienced clinician, educator or manager.

When entering the field of academia, as an inexperienced researcher, the new academic experiences heavy teaching loads and considerable pressure to pursue further education to consolidate their place within the academy. Most commonly, they are expected to obtain a doctoral qualification and build a track record of obtaining research grants and publishing scholarly papers.

Because paramedicine is still a relatively new or emerging health discipline, the new academic faces other obstacles to progressing their research careers. Internally, these barriers include academic systems that are designed for established disciplines, a lack of mentors, limited funding sources, and a poor understanding of our discipline. Externally, emerging paramedicine researchers contend with an occupational culture that until relatively recently could be described as 'anti-intellectual' and sometimes hostile to the transition of paramedic education from vocational training to university education [6]. Part of the role of the expert paramedicine researcher is to support and develop these new entrants into academic paramedicine.

With the recent growth and development of the paramedicine discipline, you are likely to see senior paramedicine academics, who may or may not be professors, in a wide range of positions and roles. While typically these roles and responsibilities are evident in position advertisements and descriptions, other Pro Bono activities are less obvious as they involve contributions to professional bodies and expert contributions to less fortunate communities, regions, or countries.

Motivations for Pursuing a Research Career

The motivations that lead our three expert researchers, and other paramedics into being researchers, varies according to their experiences within the profession. When looking at key drivers for pursuing a research career, our three expert international researchers made the following, in some cases, simple comments:

> *"To understand and explore effectiveness and efficiency of paramedic and ambulance service care"*
>
> Case Study 15

> *"An upside-down ambulance in the middle of the street began my research career. I was the department head and responded to the scene to find my vehicle in pieces. When a literature search showed that nobody had a way to prevent these events, I decided to pursue the answers."*
>
> Case Study 14

> *"I decided that I needed to understand factors that may influence the management of a patient's pain, and I strongly believed that if I could answer these questions, I could improve the patient experience."*
>
> Case Study 13

As we can see from their responses, they all took up research to get the answers to a situation that confronted or interested them. If we look at why expert researchers are involved in research, it is to get the answer(s) to a problem/issue/concern to improve clinical practice, management decision-making, policy, and paramedicine education.

Department Leadership

The role of an expert researcher in academic and paramedicine organisations brings with it additional responsibilities such as leadership roles due to their time in the organisation and experience gained over that time. Additional roles may include course co-ordination, chairing departmental and universities committees, a variety of panels related to student performance and staff progression. They might also be members of boards and committees of other associated entities like health services, professional associations and colleges.

Leading research teams is a common responsibility held by expert researchers, where they are often expected to be leaders in their field and/or have some specialist expertise in methodology, which they can then leverage with their industry networks to establish research partnerships that will facilitate external research funding. They are also expected to undertake a multitude of other tasks including writing research grant applications and associated proposals to build the research infrastructure of their institution. There is an expectation that they review the grant applications and journal articles of other researchers both nationally and internationally, mentor up and coming researchers and ensure that the intended research objectives, budgetary targets and research outcomes are successfully met. Another responsibility of the expert researcher is the important role of supervising and examining graduate research students at their own university or at other institutions both locally and internationally.

They are often expected to undertake and embrace editorial roles on journals and book ventures, writing policy commentaries, sitting on boards of management, participating as members of their professional bodies, as well as being involved in the development of policy and practice for paramedicine organisations. It is not unusual for an expert paramedicine researcher to have contact with other researchers and professional colleagues across multiple time zones during their working week.

Academia

Expert researchers in academic institutions are normally at the associate professor or professor level. Typically, in research-orientated universities and associated research institutions, appointment to these levels is dependent on an ability to demonstrate significant grant income from government and non-government organisations, a strong track record of publishing high-quality academic articles in international peer-reviewed journals with >50% in Q1 journals for associate professor and >70% for professor level. They also need to demonstrate a significant number of higher degree research (HDR), PhD/masters, completions, and others currently under supervision. Another important yardstick is peer recognition nationally for associate professors and internationally for those at the professorial level.

Associate professors and professors are expected, as part of the position they hold, to spend more time on research and research supervision compared to teaching and service. There is often an expectation that they will attract enough research funds to cover the cost of their salary or at least the research assistants that work under them on various research projects.

Benefits of Pursuing a Research Career

When we looked at the benefits or rewards of pursuing a research career, our three expert researchers shared a range of responses:

Being part of a large multicentre clinical resuscitation trial, *"As predicted, we encountered much adverse publicity and sensitive issues I had to deal with as part of the team. This was without doubt the toughest, most sensitive, challenging and fulfilling experience of my career as it built on our ability to conduct large scale resuscitation trials, resulted in very high-quality evidence, which will ultimately lead to better understanding and delivery of care for patients."*

Case Study 15

"... it is the thought that I might be a good inspiration for others; seeing students succeed, for example, is one of those rewarding moments."

Case Study 14

> *"The greatest reward has been the opportunity to contribute to the knowledge base underpinning paramedic practice, so that this can inform practice and improve the care of those in the communities we serve."*
>
> Case Study 13

These responses from expert paramedicine researchers are broad, but when you look further, their rewards are largely about bringing change to various aspects of the profession and how it functions, developing junior researchers or acting as a mentor to up and coming researchers, and inspiring others, such as undergraduate students, to get involved in research.

Why Is It Important to Engage with Experienced Paramedicine Researchers?

Providing a clear and obtainable career path for paramedicine researchers from novice to expert is an important goal for the profession at regional, national, and international levels. Without such a career structure that includes potential leadership roles, current researchers will inevitably move to other domains of practice or leave the discipline altogether [7]. Losing our best and brightest from continuing to contribute to research would be a tragedy for the profession.

Losing our future expert researchers would stymie efforts to professionalise paramedicine through the creation of our own body of knowledge/evidence, inhibit regulatory reform and self-regulation, damage the efforts of paramedicine organisations to modernise, and crucially it would take away our capacity to have a voice of our own when our profession's future is discussed and debated. In several countries, regulatory and professional bodies have recognised the importance of research capacity to the modernisation of paramedicine services and the professionalisation of the discipline through their inclusion of research knowledge and skills within paramedicine professional capability or competency expectations [8–11].

Related to this is the role that expert paramedicine researchers have in enabling the future leaders of paramedicine services and the discipline as a whole to undertake the emerging roles such a directors of paramedicine and chief paramedic positions. While many jurisdictional ambulance services internationally have medical oversight with at least one medical doctor directing clinical practice, now is arguably the time for the experienced paramedicine researcher, who has a clinical-based PhD, to be at the helm of the clinical practice direction which is based on paramedicine-driven research. Paramedics who have worked in the clinical setting, gained years of experience, and then transitioned into research, are well placed to understand the clinical environment and the research needed to progress it further. We are now seeing these types of roles in UK-based ambulance services and more recently in two Australian jurisdictions [12].

While still evolving, the UK College of Paramedics career structure is an important step toward developing the domain of research and scholarship [9]. Currently there are still comparatively few expert paramedicine researchers actively pursuing research activities, with many competent and proficient researchers herded into administrative positions within universities and organisations before they can develop into expert researchers because of limited opportunities and lack of recognition.

Being an expert researcher is 'the product of years of deliberate practice and coaching, not of any innate talent or skill' [13]. Consistently and overwhelmingly, the evidence shows that experts are always made, not born, as K. Anders Ericsson, Swedish psychologist and expert on the psychology of expertise and human performance, states [13]:

> *"The journey to truly superior performance is neither for the faint of heart nor for the impatient. The development of genuine expertise requires struggle, sacrifice, and honest, often painful self-assessment. There are no shortcuts. It will take you at least a decade to achieve expertise, and you will need to invest that time wisely, by engaging in "deliberate" practice—practice that focuses on tasks beyond your current level of competence and comfort. You will need a well-informed coach not only to guide you through deliberate practice but also to help you learn how to coach yourself. Above all, if you want to achieve top performance as a manager and a leader, you've got to forget the folklore about genius that makes many people think they cannot take a scientific approach to developing expertise. We are here to help you explode those myths"* [13].

Challenges of Pursuing a Research Career

In order to better understand the experiences of expert researchers, we asked about the challenges that they personally faced. When we look at the challenges that face researchers, across the board, but specifically for our expert paramedic researchers, the following were raised:

> *"Influencing others on the need for research and evidence-based decision making in paramedic and ambulance services practice, policy and decision making."*
>
> Case Study 15

> *"The greatest challenge was the failure of a grant funded research project early in my career. In retrospect it was a highly ambitious project."*
>
> Case Study 13

> *"The prime challenge, of course, is funding."*
>
> Case Study 14

It is interesting that the responses from these three expert paramedicine researchers all indicate that one of the main challenges in all research endeavours is the availability of funding to undertake the research. Most competitive funding bodies require the research teams to be a mix of experienced and non-experienced researchers, with the team able to demonstrate a long-standing collaboration, a track record of research project completions and dissemination of the findings which have changed practice or policy. These collaborations take time to build, obtain sufficient funding, and demonstrate research project completion and dissemination of the findings in high-quality peer-reviewed journals and presentations at prestigious international conferences. Over time, these collaborations must demonstrate that their research translates to practice, that is, changes in clinical practice, management processes, policy, and paramedicine education.

Every experienced researcher has a story of a research project that didn't go to plan. Something, somewhere during many projects fail or do not go as they theoretically should have as identified in the developmental stage. As experience builds you learn from each project you participate in or lead, all of which will help future research projects in areas such as budgeting, time frames for data collection, and understanding that reliance on external people to deliver by a certain time rarely works. You need a contingency plan for most parts of all projects.

Understanding what is possible with allocated funds and the funder's timeline comes with experience and a knowledge of processes within the project, as well as strategies to deal with deviations from the process. Finishing the project on time and on budget is the difficult part, getting all the different parts to line up and how to work around deviations takes experience, which all takes time to accumulate.

Top Tips from Expert Researchers

As a researcher you need to develop resilience, while constantly facing grant application rejections, manuscript rejections, harsh criticism from internal and external sources, and something going wrong within your project. You learn, you move on, you gain experience over the journey to help succeed in future research projects.

You need a mentor to guide and advise you on your research journey, the journey is seldom smooth, it is often rough, you feel out of your depth, and you feel like you are going round in circles and not progressing. Some poignant words from a mentor will help you see the light at the end of the tunnel and what you consider is a rough road is really a road with a few small speed humps.

> *"... I would suggest that research is a collaborative, but tough enterprise. Be prepared for a lot of rejection and critique and embrace it to make you and your work stronger. Keep patients at the centre and keep going."*
>
> Case Study 15

> *"My main tip for those embarking on a research journey is to find a mentor who can help navigate the many obstacles that lie ahead."* and ... *"make sure you choose to research a topic you are passionate about, and ask for help at an early stage."*
>
> Case Study 13

> *"... keep climbing the mountain, keep putting one foot in front of the other and keep going."* and *"The other thing I have learned is that some of the worst things that I experienced led to some of the best things that I have experienced, so don't let bad things stop you."*
>
> Case Study 14

Future Direction

As you gain knowledge and experience over time, the expectation is that you 'give back' to the up-and-coming researchers by mentoring them, reviewing junior researcher's grant applications and manuscripts. You are expected to be on journal boards as an associate or deputy editor, and eventually an editor-in-chief, all the time reviewing manuscripts in your area of expertise for multiple journals. The expectation continues where you take up leadership roles in professional colleges to promote and further the profession. Essentially, you are seen as a leader and the expectation is that you will provide the leadership for the next generation of up-and-coming researchers. As an expert researcher, you are expected to supervise honours students, master's students and PhD candidates, to extend and deepen the profession's knowledge base.

Chapter Summary

In summary, expert researchers are those who have put in the hard yards over many years and learnt by experience, often with minimal support. They have developed resilience to rejection, harsh criticism from internal and external sources, and things not going as planned within research projects. Once paramedicine researchers have reached expert status, they are expected to be leaders and mentors of emerging researchers and to promote research to paramedicine students at all levels.

Developing and supporting expert paramedicine researchers is essential to the profession for a multitude of reasons. The prime reason is that as a profession we need to keep developing the next generation of researchers to continually improve the paramedicine profession and inform the direction the profession takes through the creation of our own body of knowledge that gives a voice to paramedicine on behalf of our patients and communities.

Case Studies

As part of the research for this chapter, we asked a selection of expert researchers to respond to some key questions to reflect on their journey towards expert status. For example, where they started, key turning points, and specific experiences that shaped their journey.

Case Study 13

Name: William (Bill) Lord AM

Job title: Adjunct Professor

Affiliation(s): Monash University Department of Paramedicine

Short biography of your career.
I have worked as a paramedic for over 40 years, deciding to specialise in education early in my career. I was appointed as a lecturer in the first paramedic entry-to-practice program at an Australian university, which is where I developed an understanding of the importance of research in building the domain-specific knowledge required to support the emerging profession of paramedicine. I had few research skills at this time but was fortunate to have a head of school who supported my desire to answer questions about practice through appropriate research methods. My initial attempts were beset by failures due to my inexperience. Although disappointing at the time, these experiences taught me a lot about research design and the need to clearly communicate the need for the research to those I was trying to recruit to undertake observational studies. It is critical to clearly explain the rational and ensure that you have addressed any concerns.

Key motivators for pursuing a research career.
When working in a clinical role, I was often dismayed at paramedics' attitudes to the assessment of pain and the administration of analgesia. I often witnessed reticence to administer analgesia or accept the patient's report of

pain. I decided that I needed to understand factors that may influence the management of a patient's pain, and I strongly believed that if I could answer these questions, I could improve the patient experience.

A specific challenge you have faced pursuing and undertaking this stage of your career.
The greatest challenge was the failure of a grant-funded research project early in my career. In retrospect, it was a highly ambitious project. Although I had recruited an experienced co-researcher with expertise in the field of interest, my lack of project management skills and naive belief that paramedics would embrace the opportunity to recruit patients for this study resulted in the need to abandon the research. I'm still unsure how I managed to attract a competitive grant given my lack of research experience. This taught me much about project management, conflict resolution, dealing with multiple ethics committees, and the need for knowledge of the principles of clinical research. It's recognised that failure has the potential to provide powerful learning opportunities if we are willing to reflect on the causes, including gaps in our abilities. This experience was no exception.

Benefits/rewards of pursuing a career in research.
The greatest reward has been the opportunity to contribute to the knowledge base underpinning paramedic practice, so that this can inform practice and improve the care of those in the communities we serve. This has emerged

(continued)

(continued)

from involvement in multiple studies that span several fields of practice. As my interest in patient outcomes developed, I began to appreciate the importance of understanding the patients' perspectives of the care they receive from paramedics. I have been fortunate to be a supervisor of students who have undertaken doctoral studies into aspects of the patient experience, and the results have been enlightening. I encourage paramedics to consider specialisation in a research role. The future development of the profession depends on paramedic-led research to answer yet unanswered questions about aspects of practice that include clinical, operational, system design, and management.

Future plans and top tips/advice to others considering a career in research.
At this stage of my career, I would like to continue to act as a research mentor for students undertaking or planning to undertake research.

My main tip for those embarking on a research journey is to find a mentor who can help navigate the many obstacles that lie ahead. Professional associations have an important role in connecting members with suitable supervisors. I also strongly recommend targeted research training in the methods you are considering. For example, if your interests lie in clinical research consider completing a graduate certificate or diploma in clinical research. Preferably do this before you enrol in a higher degree in research. Although universities may include research methods coursework in a master's-level research program, you may find that this doesn't provide sufficient emphasis on the quantitative or qualitative methods that suit your study. Lastly, make sure you choose to research a topic you are passionate about, and ask for help at an early stage.

Case Study 14

Name: Brian Maguire

Job title: Senior Epidemiologist | Adjunct Professor

Affiliation(s): Leidos | Central Queensland University

Short biography of your career.
Witnessing a tragic injury when I was 17 led me to learn about how to help injured people. For about the next 20 years, I worked as a New York City paramedic. The same inspiration led me to become an instructor, so I could help others to provide care, and to leadership, so that I could develop systems to support emergency care. I did a master's degree with the intent of pursuing a career as a hospital administrator, but soon had an opportunity to become an assistant professor at the George Washington University. That led to a doctoral degree in public health. Almost as soon as I graduated, I was awarded a Fulbright scholarship to conduct research in Australia; that led to a wonderful seven-year adventure. I abruptly returned from Australia to the United States due to a family medical

(continued)

(continued)

emergency but soon found an exciting position as the senior epidemiologist at the Naval Submarine Medical Research Laboratory in Connecticut.

Key motivators for pursuing a research career.
An upside–down ambulance in the middle of the street began my research career. I was the department head and responded to the scene to find my vehicle in pieces. When a literature search showed that nobody had a way to prevent these events, I decided to pursue the answers.

A specific challenge you have faced pursuing and undertaking this stage of your career.
The prime challenge, of course, is funding. The solution, regrettably, is to instead of pursuing research that no one will fund, you pursue research that can get funded. Sadly, for our profession, that can mean doing research that is not focused on our profession.

Benefits/rewards of pursuing a career in research.
Beyond being happy every time I pay my bills, there was one year I presented in 10 countries; that was rewarding. Perhaps mostly though it is the thought that I might be a good inspiration for others; seeing students succeed, for example, is one of those rewarding moments.

Future plans and top tips/advice to others considering a career in research.
I feel like my life has been about climbing mountains. That is, I had a goal (e.g., do a master's degree) and climbed

that mountain. When I got to the top, there were many other mountains I had not seen before. Each one I climbed led me to a place where there were many new mountains. My next mountain is a new type of research project I am working on. I have to share two pieces of advice. One, keep climbing the mountain, keep putting one foot in front of the other, and keep going. The other thing I have learned is that some of the worst things that I experienced led to some of the best things that I have experienced, so don't let bad things stop you.

Case Study 15

Name: Nigel Rees

Job title: Assistant Director of Research and Innovation | Visiting Professor

Affiliation(s): Welsh Ambulance Services NHS Trust | Warwick University Medical School Clinical Trials Unit

Short biography of your career.
I joined the ambulance service in 1989 as a cadet at age sixteen. Since this time, I have engaged in part-time study, which included the Ambulance Service Institute (ASI) examinations before paramedic degree opportunities, then BSc, MSc, and PhD. I have held several clinical and leadership roles including EMT, paramedic, and

(continued)

(continued)

advanced paramedic practitioner working in the emergency department. I am also former Wales Council Member for College of Paramedics. Throughout this time, I have reflected upon the limited evidence base and fragility of knowledge in our field, which has influenced the interest in further enquiry through research.

I have been lucky to have had many good mentors and support networks to inspire me, which includes family, friends, ambulance trainers, university lecturers, and senior research and health leaders. I have been principal or chief investigator on large trials and research projects and collaborated on over £15m in research funding. I am a Fellow of College of Paramedics, Visiting Professor for Warwick University, and published 103 peer-reviewed articles. I represent WAST at research and innovation director level, sitting on many grant panels, strategy, and policy groups at local, government, national, and international level. I was awarded the Queens Ambulance Medal in 2017 New Years Honours.

Key motivators for pursuing a research career.
To understand and explore effectiveness and efficiency of paramedic and ambulance service care. An example includes struggling to reconcile complex issues related to caring for people who self-harm. Some motivations are outlined in a paper published on reflections on paramedic praxis (Rees 2021). In Ancient Greek, 'praxis' (πρᾶξις) described an activity involving free people engaging in practical reasoning leading to wise action. Praxis is driven by the moral disposition to act truly and rightly where a practical emphasis is placed on the end goal of action.

A specific challenge you have faced pursuing and undertaking this stage of your career.

Influencing others on the need for research and evidence-based decision-making in paramedic and ambulance services practice, policy, and decision-making. This has been a long and collaborative journey with many local and international colleagues. We know that research active practitioners and organisations are more efficient and effective, but vast amounts of funding and mental energies in ambulance services are misdirected into other areas, which represents a constant challenge. This will continue to be both an opportunity and threat to the paramedic profession, as such tensions I suppose have been around for a very long time and described by Plato in the Philosopher King and allegory of the cave.

Benefits/rewards of pursuing a career in research.

I was the WAST Principal Investigator for the PARA-MEDIC 2 Trial and part of the central research team. Having attempted resuscitation on many people throughout my career and having an appreciation of the research evidence in this area which is sparse, I was committed to the need for the trial. As predicted, we encountered much adverse publicity and sensitive issues I had to deal with as part of the team. This was without doubt the toughest, most sensitive, challenging, and fulfilling experience of my career as it built on our ability to conduct large-scale resuscitation trials, resulted in very high-quality evidence, which will ultimately lead to better understanding and delivery of care for patients.

(continued)

(continued)

Future plans and top tips/advice to others considering a career in research.

Given the length of time high-quality research takes to develop and deliver, I appreciate the need to focus my limited time left on leading and supporting the development and delivery of high-quality research in our sector. This will include leading future high-quality research, developing policy and strategy, peer and scientific review of research papers and grant applications, and providing support for the development of others who are pursuing a research career.

In terms of advice, I would suggest that research is a collaborative but tough enterprise. Be prepared for a lot of rejection and critique and embrace it to make you and your work stronger. Keep patients at the centre and keep going.

References

1. Scholz, O.R. (2009). Experts: what they are and how we recognize them – a discussion of Alvin Goldman's views. *Grazer Philosophische Studien* 79 (1): 187–205.
2. Croce, M. (2018). On what it takes to be an expert. *The Philosophical Quarterly* 69 (274): 1–21.
3. Reed, B., Cowin, L., O'Meara, P., and Wilson, I. (2019). Professionalism and professionalisation in the discipline of paramedicine. *Australasian Journal of Paramedicine* 16: 1–10.
4. Munro, G.G., O'Meara, P., and Mathisen, B. (2019). Paramedic transition into an academic role in universities: a qualitative survey of paramedic academics in Australia and New Zealand. *Irish Journal of Paramedicine* 4 (1): 1–11.

5. Simpson, P., Barr, N., Reid, D. et al. (2023). Profiling the Australasian paramedicine tertiary academic sector and workforce: a cross-sectional study. *Paramedicine* 20 (6): 206–213.

6. Maguire, B.J., Maniscalco, P.M., Gerard, D.R. et al. (2024). *Creating the Emergency Medical Services System of the Future: the role of the EMS Education Agenda.* USA: Verizon https://downloads.regulations.gov/NHTSA-2023-0037-0101/attachment_1.pdf.

7. O'Meara, P. and Maguire, B. (2018). Developing a sustainable academic workforce in paramedicine. *Australian Universities' Review* 60 (1): 54–56.

8. Cameron, C. and Batt, A.M. (2024). *PAC Career Framework for Paramedics.* Ottawa: Paramedic Association of Canada.

9. College of Paramedics. Paramedic Career Framework London 2023. 5th. https://collegeofparamedics.co.uk/COP/ProfessionalDevelopment/post_reg_career_framework.aspx.

10. Paramedic Board of Australia (2021). Professional Capabilities For Registered Paramedics. In: Australian Health Practitioner Regulation Agency, editor. Canberra.

11. Makrides, T., Ross, L., Gosling, C. et al. (2022). Defining two novel sub models of the Anglo-American paramedic system: a Delphi study. *Australasian Emergency Care* 25 (3): 229–234.

12. Australasian College of Paramedicine (2021). https://paramedics.org/storage/news/Chief-Paramedic-Officers-Position-Statement-AUS.pdf.

13. Ericsson, K., Prietula, M., and Cokely, E. (2007). *The Making of an Expert.* Brighton, MA: Harvard Business Review https://hbr.org/2007/07/the-making-of-an-expert.

Section 3

Expert Advice

Chapter 8

Expert Advice

Julia Williams
Department of Paramedic Science, University of Hertfordshire, Hatfield, United Kingdom

Chapter Objectives

By the end of this chapter, you will be able to:

1. Understand the importance of mentorship in research career development.
2. Recognise the usefulness of collaboration and networking in building a successful research career.

Research-focused Careers for Paramedics, First Edition.
Edited by Gregory A. Whitley and Scott Munro.
© 2025 John Wiley & Sons Ltd. Published 2025 by John Wiley & Sons Ltd.

3. Identify common challenges in a research career and develop strategies to address them.
4. Reflect on your approaches for writing effective funding applications.
5. Apply stage-specific advice to navigate different phases of a research career.
6. Integrate insights from experienced researchers to strengthen grant applications for clinical academic development.

Introduction

In the rapidly evolving landscape of health and social care, the roles of paramedic researchers are in the forefront. Recognised as a pillar of practice in the College of Paramedics' Career Framework [1] for several years, opportunities for paramedics to work in research continue to increase in a variety of roles. The development of clinical academics in our profession is still in early stages, although, as discussed earlier in this book (**Chapter 1**), there is still some inconsistency in how we define these terms. In my interpretation, at one level, clinical academics bridge the gap between clinical practice and research, working to translate scientific advancements into improved patient outcomes. However, definitions can vary among individuals and organisations.

Pursuing a career as a paramedic researcher is both challenging and deeply rewarding [2, 3] often forming part of the broader work of a clinical academic. It requires not only a dedication to clinical excellence but also a commitment to rigorous scientific inquiry. There are many reasons why people undertake research pathways in their career development. Some individuals may have deliberately chosen to focus on paramedic research, mapping out a series of well-defined steps from novice researcher to potential consultant, director or professorial roles. Others might have started with a single research experience, perhaps as a student research intern or as a research paramedic on a specific study, and discovered a growing interest in research but they do not necessarily want research to be their sole focus. The College of Paramedics [4] refers to this as the 'portfolio paramedic', where individuals develop diverse roles within their career. For example, in my own case, I've specialised in research but remained active in teaching and learning in paramedicine and maintained clinical practice albeit not in equal proportions. While this sounds ideal in theory, there are just not enough of these opportunities currently available to meet demand within the paramedic workforce, and we are not always able to source roles that facilitate working across all four pillars of practice. However, this is not just unique to paramedicine as similar difficulties are found in other health and social care professions [5]. Encouragingly, these opportunities are becoming more common place, but there is still a long way to go.

As with any resource, this chapter has its limitations—what you find here are suggestions drawn from my own learning and experiences, and one chapter alone can't cover everything. I have chosen to present it in a form of question and answers (see **Table 8.1** for the list of questions), based on actual questions that people have asked me during my years as a professor within our professional communities of research practice. I suggest you reflect on what's useful and appropriate for you, supplement it with other sources, and apply it in ways that fit your unique path.

Table 8.1   List of questions

Question

Research as a career choice
What are the different ways to get into paramedic research?
What advice do you have for those who are already on their way on a research pathway, particularly at MSc or doctoral level?
How does the focus change for postdoctoral researchers?

The role of mentoring
Mentorship seems like a recurring theme. How important is mentorship in a research career?
What should I look for in a mentor, and how can I build a productive mentor—mentee relationship?
Is it beneficial to have multiple mentors?

The power of networking
How does one build an effective professional network?
Social media is also a networking tool nowadays. Do you have advice on using it effectively?

Crafting effective funding applications
Can you elaborate on the funding landscape for research and any tips for new researchers seeking grants?
Securing funding sounds essential, but it also seems like a challenge. How can researchers craft effective funding applications?
What's the first step in writing a strong application?
I have heard of the three 'Ps' in research funding: Can you explain these?
Any final thoughts on what makes a successful application?

Overcoming common challenges
Research careers come with unique challenges. How do you balance clinical and research responsibilities?
Setbacks and rejections are common in research. How do you handle them?
Getting published can be a real challenge: what are your top tips?

Whether you are just beginning your journey, seeking to establish research independence, or transitioning into a research leadership role, I hope the advice and insights in this chapter serve as a valuable guide to help you to embrace the challenges, leverage the opportunities, and let your passion for research and clinical excellence drive you towards achieving your professional goals.

Research as a Career Choice

Question*: What are the different ways to get into paramedic research?*

My Response: There are many routes into research. Some people actively plan their research career, while others might end up in research almost by accident. For instance, they might take on a position as a study-specific research paramedic focussing mainly on research delivery of an existing study to gain hands-on experience in research. These roles are becoming more common, especially in ambulance services in the United Kingdom as we undertake large-scale trials like PARAMEDIC 3 [6] for example.

Opportunities are emerging all the time, so it's worth talking to other paramedic researchers to see what options might suit you. Some countries have government-funded career development awards targeted from novice clinical researchers all the way to expert clinical researchers.

If you want to move forward in research, then just like any other extended scope role, you need to achieve additional knowledge and skills. When you are just starting out, focus on developing skills in research methodologies and data analysis and look to gain practical experience of working in research. It is useful to find a mentor to guide you through these early stages. Networking is also essential, so attend research conferences and join paramedic professional bodies, who should have a variety of research resources to support you. Remember there are also non-paramedic groups that can help, such as Special Interest Groups; broader healthcare professional communities, such as Emergency Medicine groups, and specialist methods groups.

Question: What advice do you have for those who are already on their way on a research pathway, particularly at MSc or doctoral level?

My Response: At MSc or doctoral level, the focus should be on building a strong research foundation. I like to think of it as cultivating the roots of a tree; strong roots will support growth and resilience. Similarly to novice researchers, it's essential to further develop skills in research methodologies, data analysis, and academic writing. If you haven't found a mentor yet, take the time to explore who might be available. Having someone in this role early in your journey can provide the guidance, feedback, and support that are essential for your professional growth.

Keep building your network and connecting with peers and senior researchers. Utilise resources like *Paramedic PhD* [7] and the *McNally Project* [8] which can help you identify researchers worldwide who are engaged in similar work. Additionally, explore the College of Paramedics Research Database—*CReD* [9]. This international directory helps minimise research duplication and fosters networking within research communities.

Publishing your research in peer-reviewed journals is a key milestone that boosts your credibility, enhances your professional profile, and is vital at this stage of your research career. Additionally, make sure to register for ORCID [10], a free service that provides a unique identifier for researchers. This tool supports networking, increases the visibility of your work, and offers many other advantages throughout your career.

Question: How does the focus change for postdoctoral researchers?

My Response: Postdoctoral researchers are aiming to establish independence and a unique research identity. At this stage, it's important to take the lead on your own research projects and pursue independent funding opportunities. Interdisciplinary collaboration is also key as working with researchers from other disciplines can add breadth and impact to your research. Consistently managing projects and publishing your work is essential, along with creating a comprehensive career development plan that outlines both short- and long-term goals. Collaborating with a mentor can be especially valuable for planning your next steps and shaping a clear career trajectory.

It's equally important to start focusing on research leadership. Nurturing the next generation of researchers is essential. Just as you valued mentorship (and likely still do, as having a mentor is beneficial at every career stage), newcomers to the field will also seek guidance. Consider exploring opportunities to join research leadership programmes or reaching out to local research departments and universities to offer your support as a mentor in your area of expertise. Share your knowledge and experiences with others, as this is how we collectively strengthen future research capacity and capability within our workforce.

The Role of Mentoring

Question: Mentorship seems like a recurring theme. How important is mentorship in a research career?

My Response: Mentorship is absolutely fundamental in research. A good mentor provides guidance, support, and insights based on their own experiences. It's like having a guide who helps you navigate the challenges and capitalise on opportunities. In my view, everyone in research, at any level, can benefit from a mentor.

Question: What should I look for in a mentor, and how can I build a productive mentor–mentee relationship?

My Response: Finding the right mentor depends on what you need in terms of expertise, mentoring style, or experience in your specific research area. Look for mentors with a solid track record and whose expertise aligns with your goals. It's a good idea to have an initial meeting to discuss expectations and assess if their style and availability match your needs.

A strong mentor–mentee relationship requires clear communication, mutual respect, and regular meetings. Define your goals and be proactive in updating your mentor on progress. At the same time, be open to feedback as constructive criticism is essential for growth. A good mentoring relationship is collaborative, but remember, you're ultimately responsible for your own choices.

Question: Is it beneficial to have multiple mentors?

My Response: Yes, having multiple mentors can provide a range of perspectives and expertise, especially if your research is interdisciplinary. Think of it as building a personal board of advisors. However, it's not about accumulating as many mentors as possible! It's about selecting mentors who complement each other and meet different aspects of your development needs.

The Power of Networking

Question: Let's talk about networking. How does one build an effective professional network?

My Response: Networking is a vital part of a research career, serving as a gateway to resources, collaborations, and innovative ideas. Conferences and workshops are excellent starting points, as they bring together seasoned experts and emerging researchers in a dynamic environment. Be strategic about which events you attend, focusing on those that closely align with your research interests. Whenever possible, research attendees and speakers in advance, and prepare thoughtful questions to help initiate meaningful conversations.

Joining professional organisations in your field is another effective way to stay connected with the research community. These organisations often offer exclusive networking opportunities, and as you advance in your career, taking on leadership roles within them can further strengthen and broaden your collaborations.

Question: Social media is also a networking tool nowadays. Do you have advice on using it effectively?

My Response: Social media can be a double-edged sword, and it's essential to use it effectively while maintaining control over how it influences your time and focus. There's no doubt that social media has revolutionised the way researchers connect and share their work. Individual preferences, personal values, and political beliefs often influence how and which social media platforms people choose to engage with. Platforms like LinkedIn and ResearchGate are particularly useful for discussing ideas, forming collaborations, and enabling detailed communication when needed. In contrast, platforms like X (formerly Twitter) can be more restrictive, especially for non-subscribers.

To make the most of these tools, share your work, actively engage with others by liking and commenting on their posts, and initiate respectful, concise conversations via direct messages. Social media offers a convenient way to stay updated and build connections across geographical boundaries, but I think we need to be mindful of the risks involved, such as losing time and focus. Additionally, it's easy to fall into the trap of comparing your progress to others, especially when colleagues share curated highlights of their achievements. This can lead to unnecessary pressure or feelings of inadequacy. Another challenge is navigating echo chambers, where the diversity of ideas may be limited, reinforcing pre-existing views and stifling critical thinking. To counter these issues, it's helpful to set clear goals for your social media use, follow accounts that challenge your perspectives, and periodically evaluate whether your online interactions align with your personal and professional values.

Crafting Effective Funding Applications

Question: Can you elaborate on the funding landscape for research and any tips for new researchers seeking grants?

My Response: Securing funding is highly competitive, and new researchers often face significant challenges in obtaining grants, so collaborating with experienced researchers can improve your chance of success. While government grants are a key funding source, there are also opportunities through smaller grants offered by professional bodies, as well as charities, local universities, industry partners, among others.

When applying for funding, you need to understand the funder's criteria and demonstrate both the importance and feasibility of your project. A well-structured, concise application that aligns with the funder's priorities can make a strong impression. Be sure to highlight your expertise, past achievements, and the potential impact of your research. Keep in mind that preparing a grant application is a time-intensive process that can take several months from initial planning to submission, so start early and stay organised. You may need to apply for funding that buys your time so that you can focus on and write a full funding application.

Question: Securing funding sounds essential, but it also seems like a challenge. How can researchers craft effective funding applications?

My Response: You're absolutely right—securing funding is one of the most significant challenges in a research career, and a well-prepared application can be the key to success. Crafting a successful grant application requires a strategic approach, clear communication, and a thorough understanding of the funding body's priorities. Your application should showcase your expertise and that of your team, emphasising the importance and potential impact of your research. It's essential to include a detailed and clear research plan with a well-defined methodology, timeline, and budget. Building an appropriate research grant application team with a good balance of appropriate expertise including lay/public/patient members, experience, skills, knowledge and a proven track record can be the difference between success and rejection.

There are resources available to help you develop effective grant applications. Government-funded career development awards, such as those provided by the National Institute for Health and Care Research in the United Kingdom, provide a publicly available Chair's report [11] for each round, providing valuable insights and generic tips that apply to most grant applications.

Question: *What's the first step in writing a strong application?*

My Response: The first step in securing funding is thoroughly understanding the criteria set by the funding body. Think of it like preparing for an exam—knowing exactly what the 'examiners' are looking for is advantageous. This requires more than just skimming the guidelines; it involves a deep dive into their priorities and goals. Are they focused on practical applications, theoretical advancements, or addressing specific challenges?

Present your proposal as a feasible solution to a problem the funding body cares about. Highlight how your project addresses their goals or contributes to solving a challenge in the field. *Explain why your research matters.* Reviewers want to understand the potential impact of your work—how it could advance knowledge, influence policy, or provide practical solutions. Clearly connect your project's significance to the funder's mission, showing them why it's an investment worth making.

Question: I have heard of the three 'Ps' in research funding. Can you explain these?

My Response: Sure, but I like to think of five 'Ps' in fact. These are things to think about in your application, whatever type of funding you are going for.

Person refers to the researcher's skills, experience, and professional profile. It's essential to demonstrate your research capabilities, accomplishments, and expertise, particularly when applying for a personal award or leading a grant application. For grant applications focused on individual research studies rather than personal awards, this is where you highlight the collective expertise and experience of the proposed grant team. Emphasise the team's achievements, including their successful track record with previously funded research projects.

Patient and Public Involvement and Engagement frequently referred to as 'experts by experience'. It's essential to engage and involve these individuals from the very beginning, as you assemble your application team, and to continue their involvement throughout all stages of the research. Funders want to see evidence as to how these team members shape, develop and influence the research from inception to dissemination.

Place refers to the institution where you conduct your research or the academic setting you are proposing for your study. A supportive environment with adequate resources, a strong collaborative culture, and a solid reputation can have a significant impact on your research and career development. If you're applying for a personal award, such as a studentship or fellowship, the institution's reputation and track record in successfully supporting similar awards to completion will be closely evaluated, along with the expertise and profile of your nominated supervisors.

Project emphasises the importance of an original, feasible, and impactful research proposal. Your project should be clear, innovative, and have a well-defined plan. Ensure your research proposal is feasible and realistic. You should provide a detailed research plan, including a timeline, methodology, and budget and include discussion as to any potential challenges and how you will overcome them. Remember to clearly explain how it will benefit the field, society, and possibly influence policy or practice.

Finally, **Publishing** is about sharing your research with the world. Disseminating your findings through various channels is a cornerstone of a successful academic career. It is through publications and other forms of communication that your work reaches a broader audience, enriches the collective knowledge of your field, and helps establish your reputation as a researcher. Publishing is not just a professional responsibility—it's the culmination of your research efforts. Without sharing your findings, the impact of your work is significantly diminished.

Question: Any final thoughts on what makes a successful application?

My Response: A strong funding application resonates with reviewers by appealing to both their logical and emotional perspectives. It is well-organised, technically robust, and presents a strong case for support. Taking the time to refine each section and create a clear, persuasive message can significantly increase your chances of success. Remember, reviewers often have to evaluate many applications, so making yours easy to read and understand is a major advantage.

Avoid jargon and use plain language, especially as some reviewers may not be experts in your discipline. Be succinct and ensure every sentence adds value, focusing on the significance, feasibility, or potential impact of your research. Adopt the reviewer's perspective and critically evaluate your application. Allow plenty of time to prepare your application, especially for larger grants that may require internal approvals or signatures. Don't leave submission to the last minute as unexpected delays can jeopardise your chances.

Consider inclusivity. Often, groups of people are marginalised during the conduct of clinical research, such as those with disabilities, from ethnic minority backgrounds, and children and young people, for example. Be cognisant of those whose voice may not be heard during participant recruitment and data collection and where possible, make accommodations to facilitate inclusivity.

Finally, proofread thoroughly. Review your application multiple times over several days to remove errors, improve flow, and ensure consistency. Double-check all facts, figures, and references for accuracy, and make sure the narrative is cohesive. An application filled with typographical errors or inconsistencies can detract from its professionalism and leave a poor impression on the review panel.

Summary of Top Tips for Writing a Successful Funding Application:

1. **Understand the Funding Body's Priorities:** Align your research proposal with the specific priorities and goals of the funding body.
2. **Engage with Stakeholders:** Demonstrate how your research will involve and benefit stakeholders, including patients, healthcare providers, and policymakers. This is particularly important as patient and public involvement is increasingly valued and in some instances, mandated.
3. **Build Your Application Team Early:** Include a range of appropriate people depending on what your research topic is. You should include people with track records of successful completion of research in a relevant area but there is often room to include at least one early career researcher. Include lay/public/patients/ service users/experts by experience at the beginning.
4. **Demonstrate Feasibility:** Clearly outline your research methodology and ensure it is detailed and

feasible. Include timelines, potential challenges, and mitigation strategies.

5. **Highlight Your Team's Track Record:** Showcase your previous research achievements, publications, and any prior funding you have received. This helps establish your credibility and capability as a researcher.

6. **Plan for Dissemination:** Outline your plans for disseminating your research findings. This could include publications, presentations at conferences, and engagement with media and public health bodies.

7. **Seek Feedback at an Early Stage:** Before submitting your application, seek feedback from colleagues, mentors, or previous grant reviewers. They can provide valuable insights and help identify any weaknesses in your application.

Overcoming Common Challenges

Question: Research careers come with unique challenges. How do you balance clinical and research responsibilities?

My Response: Balancing clinical and research work can feel like walking a tightrope, especially in paramedicine, where our roles as clinical academics are still developing. Effective time management and setting clear boundaries between clinical and research duties are essential.

In 2015, I created an opportunity between my university employer and an ambulance service to develop a role that allowed me to engage in both clinical practice and research. This collaboration was a turning point, as it helped establish a model that allowed me to stay active in patient care and lead research in an ambulance Trust while also dedicating meaningful time to research and teaching at the university. The position has since evolved, and I've used this experience to advocate for similar roles within the field, creating new research-focused positions that align with the College of Paramedics' Career Framework (2024).

However, securing long-term, substantive research positions in paramedicine is still challenging. Funding limitations, short-term projects, and the need to establish a permanent place for research within clinical organisations often complicate the path forward. To address this, I find it helpful to collaborate with both clinical and academic leaders to advocate for research positions that support professional growth across clinical, research, and academic settings. Collaboration and creativity have been key in designing roles that fulfil clinical needs while fostering research, so **be bold** and put business plans to your institutions if the opportunities do not already exist. Engaging with these leaders has also been a critical step in normalising research positions within paramedicine, gradually building support for dual roles within the profession, but there is a long road ahead of us to expand these opportunities.

Question: *Setbacks and rejections are common in research. How do you handle them?*

My Response: Setbacks and rejections are part of the process. Each setback is an opportunity to refine ideas, strengthen research methods, and clarify goals. For example, feedback from a rejected grant application can reveal blind spots in the proposal or identify aspects of the study that need more rigorous design. Rather than seeing rejection as a dead end, I approach it as a tool to fine-tune my research skills and improve future applications. With each piece of constructive criticism, I gain new insights into what resonates with reviewers and what needs adjusting to be successful the next time around.

Building a support network is useful in handling these challenges. Paramedic research can sometimes feel isolating, particularly if you're pioneering research within a clinical environment where your role is not yet fully understood. Connecting with colleagues who have faced similar challenges, as well as mentors who have navigated their own setbacks, provides both practical advice and emotional support. These individuals can offer strategies to move forward, share their own experiences of overcoming hurdles, and remind you that setbacks are part of a broader journey.

Finally, embracing a mindset of continuous learning and adaptability is key. Paramedic research often involves dynamic, real-world environments with variables that can shift unexpectedly. This makes flexibility an asset. Embracing the iterative nature of research strengthens my resilience and broadens my experience, as each challenge refines my skills and enhances my growth as a researcher

Question: *Getting published can be a real challenge: what are your top tips?*

My Response: Publishing can be challenging, especially for early-career researchers. Common barriers include limited experience, time constraints, and the competitive nature of academic publishing. Seek mentorship from experienced researchers who can guide you through the publishing process. Collaborate with colleagues to share knowledge and resources. As with grant writing, do not underestimate how long it can take to write a paper and allow plenty of time to get drafts of your work out to others to informally review it. Try and allocate dedicated time for writing and revising manuscripts. Treat publishing as a priority alongside your other responsibilities. You should be prepared for rejection and if it happens, then use it as an opportunity to improve your work.

Top Tips for Getting a Paper Published:

- **Choose the 'Right' Journal:** Select journals that align with your research topic and audience. Consider the journal's impact factor, readership, and acceptance rate. The journal could be topic, population, method, or discipline specific.
- **Quality Over Quantity:** Focus on producing high-quality research that makes a significant contribution to the field. Prioritise quality over quantity in your publications.
- **Clear and Concise Writing:** Write clearly and concisely, presenting your research in a logical and coherent manner. Ensure that your manuscript follows the journal's guidelines, or it will just be returned at the start of the process. Use reporting guidelines (see EQUATOR Network [12] for a wide range of resources and toolkits to assist you).

> • **Responding to Reviewers:** Engage constructively with reviewers' comments. Be open to feedback and willing to make revisions to improve your manuscript.
> • **Ethical Considerations:** Ensure that your research adheres to ethical standards, including proper citation of sources and avoiding plagiarism.

Insights into Applying for a Personal Research Award

Professor Natalie Pattison offers a behind-the-scenes look at what makes a successful funding application and candidate when you are applying for a personal research award such as a funded studentship or fellowship.

Biography and Current Role

Professor Natalie Pattison is a leading figure in clinical academic research in the United Kingdom who has worked clinically in cancer, critical care and critical care outreach. She holds several key leadership positions, including:

- Chair of the National Outreach Forum
- Deputy Lead for the National Institute of Health and Care Research (NIHR) National Specialty Group for Critical Care
- Board member (co-opted) of the Intensive Care Society Council and the Critical Care Leadership Forum
- Reviewer for national and international grant panels
- Member of the NIHR Doctoral Clinical and Practitioner Academic Fellowship (DCAF) funding panel

With her extensive experience of supervising clinical academics, Professor Pattison provides invaluable insights into what makes a successful funding application for advancing a clinical academic research career.

What Is a Personal Research Award?

A personal research award, or fellowship, is funding to undertake a programme of training and development. It may involve the acquisition of an academic qualification, such as a master's or doctoral degree. They often fund the applicant's salary, course fees (for those doing academic qualifications), research costs, and costs for training and development (short courses and research visits, etc.).

A research grant, on the other hand, only funds the research costs and staff salary time.

What a Strong Funding Application Should Include

According to Professor Pattison, strong funding applications for clinical academic research careers share several key characteristics. Person, project, and place are often cited as key. Applicants not only need to clearly articulate the research question, its significance, and demonstrate robust methodology but also outline the future potential of that individual as a clinical or research leader, as well as discuss where they work and how they will be supported as a clinical academic. Successful applications demonstrate the feasibility of the research and the investigator's ability to execute the project. Additionally, these applications align well with national priorities and address important gaps in current knowledge or practice.

1. **Clear and Compelling Narrative:** A strong application tells a compelling story. It begins with a well-defined research question that addresses a significant gap or need in clinical practice. The narrative should flow logically, making a convincing case for why the research is important and how it will be conducted.
2. **Robust Methodology:** The methodology section should be detailed and robust, demonstrating that the research plan is feasible and well thought out. This includes clear descriptions of the study design, data collection methods, analysis plans, and timelines.
3. **Significance and Impact:** Successful applications highlight the potential impact of the research on patient care, policy, or advancing clinical practice. Demonstrating the relevance of the research to clinical priorities and its potential to improve health outcomes is crucial as is involvement of experts by experience in the designing of the research.
4. **Investigator Credentials and Organisational Support:** Strong applications showcase the investigator's expertise, previous research achievements, and capacity to carry out the proposed study. This can be supported by a strong track record of publications (ideally with some first author publications), previous grants or awards, and relevant clinical experience. There must be a robust statement of organisational support that demonstrates how the applicant will be supported through their research award (and beyond).

Common Pitfalls

Professor Pattison notes several common pitfalls that applicants should avoid:

1. **Poorly Defined Research Questions:** Lack of a focused research question often fails to convince reviewers of the value.
2. **Vague Methodologies:** Applications that are vague or lacking in methodological detail can raise concerns about the feasibility and reliability of the proposed research.
3. **Lack of Alignment:** Applications that do not align well with the funding body's priorities or fail to address important gaps in the field are less likely to be successful.
4. **Overambitious Plans:** While ambition is important, overambitious research plans that are not realistic within the given time frame and resources can be detrimental.
5. **Insufficient Preliminary Data:** Providing preliminary data or robust literature reviews can strengthen the application.

Key Points from Professor Pattison

Professor Pattison emphasises the importance of clarity and coherence in applications. Reviewers need to quickly see the significance of the research, alongside value for money. Clear objectives, a well-structured methodology, and a strong justification for the proposed study are critical components that reviewers look for.

Chapter Summary

This chapter serves as a practical guide for paramedics pursuing a career focussed on research, offering advice and insights to support their journey. The content explores essential components of building a successful research career, emphasising the importance of networking, mentorship, and suggesting effective strategies for tackling common research challenges. A career in paramedic research opens up a world of opportunities for those with a curious mind. While it demands a commitment to learning, adaptability, and the willingness to embrace uncertainty, the rewards are great.

References

1. College of Paramedics (2024). *Paramedic Career Framework,* 5th Edition Revised. Bridgwater, UK: College of Paramedics.
2. McClelland, G., Limmer, M., and Charlton, K. (2023). The RESearch PARamedic Experience (RESPARE) study: a qualitative study exploring the experiences of research paramedics working in the United Kingdom. *British Paramedic Journal* 7 (4): 14–22.
3. Runacres, J., Harvey, H., O'Brien, S., and Halck, A. (2024). Paramedics as researchers: A systematic review of paramedic perspectives of engaging in research activity from training to practice. *The Journal of Emergency Medicine* 66 (6): e680–e689.
4. College of Paramedics (2024). Portfolio paramedics. https://collegeofparamedics.co.uk/COP/Become_a_Paramedic/Portfolio_Paramedic/COP/ProfessionalDevelopment/Portfolio%20Paramedic.aspx?hkey=cd839df9-c508-4c0c-9b72-07d1c8abef71 (accessed 3 September 2024).
5. Dhillo, W. (2024). How we can support research careers for health and social care professionals. National Institute of Health and Care Research. www.nihr.ac.uk/blog/how-we-can-support-

research-careers-health-and-social-care-professionals (accessed 6 August 2024).

6. Couper, K., Ji, C., Deakin, C.D. et al. (2024). A randomized trial of drug route in out-of-hospital cardiac arrest. *The New England Journal of Medicine* 392 (4): 336–348. https://doi.org/10.1056/NEJMoa2407780.

7. Paramedic PhD. www.paramedicphd.com (accessed 8 June 2024).

8. McNally project. http://mcnallyproject.ca/ (accessed 15 November 2024).

9. College of Paramedics (2024). Research studies database. College of Paramedics. https://research.collegeofparamedics.co.uk (accessed 1 May 2024).

10. Open Researcher and Contributor ID (ORCID) (2024). About ORCID. ORCID. https://orcid.org (accessed 6 May 2024).

11. National Institute for Health and Care Research (NIHR) (2024). DCAF Chair's report. National Institute for Health and Care Research. https://www.nihr.ac.uk/nihr-doctoral-clinical-practitioner-and-academic-fellowship-dcaf-chairs-report-round-4 (accessed 7 November 2024).

12. Enhancing the Quality and Transparency of Health Research (EQUATOR) Network (2024). One stop shop for writing and publishing high-impact health research. EQUATOR. https://equator-network.org (accessed 1 June 2024).

Index

Note: Page numbers in *italics* refer to figures and *t* refer to tables.

Research-focused Careers for Paramedics, First Edition.
Edited by Gregory A. Whitley and Scott Munro.
© 2025 John Wiley & Sons Ltd. Published 2025 by John Wiley & Sons Ltd.

Printed and bound by CPI Group (UK) Ltd, Croydon, CR0 4YY

30/06/2025

14695991-0001